Body-First Healing

Body-First Healing

Get Unstuck and Recover from Trauma with Somatic Healing

Brittany Piper

AVERY

an imprint of Penguin Random House

New York

AVERY

an imprint of Penguin Random House LLC
1745 Broadway, New York, NY 10019
penguinrandomhouse.com

Library of Congress Cataloging-in-Publication Data is on file.
Hardcover ISBN: 9780593718650
eBook ISBN: 9780593718667

Printed in the United States of America
1st Printing

Book design by Ashley Tucker

Somatic Experiencing®, SE™, SEP™, CSS™, SCOPE™, Crisis Stabilization and Safety™, the Sphere Logo®, the CSS Logos and all associated trade dress are owned by, and used with permission of Somatic Experiencing Trauma Institute ("SEI") and are registered and used in the US, Canada, EU, and other countries in English with certain foreign transliterations. The SEI marks may be used only with the express permission of SEI.

SEI does not endorse, approve, or support any specific authors, practitioners, or contributors unless explicitly stated otherwise. Views, opinions, methodologies, or practices expressed by individuals regarding SEI modalities are their own and do not necessarily reflect the official views of SEI.

The authorized representative in the EU for product safety and compliance is Penguin Random House Ireland, Morrison Chambers, 32 Nassau Street, Dublin D02 YH68, Ireland, https://eu-contact.penguin.ie.

This book is dedicated to the children found in each of us. The ones who fought to keep us free. The ones whose armor protects us still today. May they rest now. May they play. May they dream. We can take it from here.

Contents

AUTHOR'S NOTE

From Concrete Bottom to Resilience and Healing

A hero lies in you.
   —**Mariah Carey**

As I type this letter to you, my dear reader, I am sitting at my kitchen counter with my four-month-old daughter still sound asleep in her car seat beside me. We just arrived back home from running a few errands. My three-year-old son is at the park with our nanny, and my husband is upstairs in his office working. In the background, a shuffled blend of Celine Dion radio plays lightly through the house speakers, filling my quiet and sun-soaked home with echoed melodies that remind me of my childhood—Whitney Houston, Mariah Carey, and Phil Collins, to name a few.

To many, this might seem like just another boring day.

But for *younger* me, the twentysomething Britt literally battling for her life, this was the type of day I couldn't have even dreamed of—a day devoid of chaos and unhealthy behaviors in the name of survival. Perhaps you know the feeling. The juxtaposition of hopelessly longing for the never-ending roller coaster of dysfunction to stop, while also being fearfully resistant to exiting the ride you've come to know all too well.

As someone who survived and made it off that roller coaster, I'm here to tell you it doesn't have to be a life sentence. And that what will actually save you from the chaos you're held captive to isn't found outside of you but *within you*. It's true; the hero of this story isn't your therapist, your medications, your partner, your kids, or even this book. The hero in your life, as cheesy as it sounds, has and always will be . . . you. Believe it or not, your body and brain were innately and brilliantly built not just to survive in the worst of conditions, but to truly live and thrive. You, my friend, are your own best healer.

Ironically enough, as I write to you these words, Mariah Carey's self-empowering anthem "Hero" plays in the background.

Look inside you and be strong . . .

I've come to learn, in both my personal and professional lives, that healing doesn't mean becoming a new version of you. *Healing is rediscovering who you were, before the survival responses of your nervous system told you who to be.* Following trauma that's too overwhelming, the nervous system often becomes ensnared in chronic states of survival mode (fight, flight, shutdown, functional freeze, or fawn, which you will learn about in detail later in this book). This can leave us seemingly trapped in the adrenaline-fueled survival responses of the past—aka the "threat response cycle"—even though we are safely living in the present. As Dr. Peter A. Levine, the developer of the Somatic Experiencing® trauma recovery method we will explore together in this book, aptly describes it:

> *Trauma is an internal straitjacket created when a devastating moment is frozen in time. It stifles the unfolding of being and strangles our attempts to move forward with our lives. It disconnects us from ourselves, others, nature, and spirit. When overwhelmed by threat, we are frozen in fear, as though our instinctive survival energies (adrenaline) were "all dressed up with no place to go."*

With this description in mind, we can easily say that healing is aimed at allowing ourselves—more specifically, our nervous system—to get unstuck from the overwhelm of the past and catch up to the safety of the present.

Soma means "of the body," and in Somatic Experiencing (SE™), we gently guide you out of your head and into the experience of your body, where the nervous system can be accessed. By learning the language of your unique system through sensation, feeling, and emotion, you'll have a greater capacity to process discomfort or what was once too overwhelming to be with. This will allow your system to complete its thwarted threat response cycle and release the pent-up adrenaline, or survival energy, from the past. Through Somatic Experiencing, you can become a more present and regulated you.

Imagine the protective layers you've had to wear to survive trauma as a set of nesting dolls. Healing necessitates cracking open and shedding each heroic layer—the people-pleasing part of you, the anxious part of you, the defensive part of you, the isolating part of you, and the numb part of you. Healing is holding compassionate space and understanding for each of these versions of you, while also reminding yourself that the core of who you are has never been too far lost, but just hidden away under these shields that were meant to keep you safe.

Woven throughout the pages of this book, you'll witness my own confrontations with the many coats of armor that once kept me alive but eventually overstayed their welcome. You'll also be given a somatic roadmap that will take you on a profound yet gentle journey to come to know your own armor. When in your life did your nervous system armor up? Is it fight, flight, shutdown, freeze, or fawn? What are the characteristics of that armor? How does it inform your patterns of behaviors, thoughts, beliefs, emotional states, overall physical health, and more? Why, even after the trauma has passed and the battle is over, are you *stuck* with this armor on? How can you begin to slowly remove it? And what will take its place?

My deepest hope for you is that while reading this book, you begin to soften to the parts of you that you've long seen as burdensome and self-sabotaging, and recognize that they were simply maladaptive coping patterns of self-protection. I hope that by staying open and curious about these patterns, and by learning the science behind what drives them, you learn that you in fact are not broken and do not need fixing, and that the ways you've had to survive make perfect sense, based on your body's and your brain's instinctual responses and past experiences. When I reflect on my own healing, that's what I would have hoped for myself, too. This book is the culmination of everything I wish I had known in my darkest years. This is translation work, really, not the discovery of new information. It's the simple somatic practices, the revolutionary knowledge, the inspiration, and the compassion that would have gifted me a lot more living and a lot less just surviving.

If you're reading this book, it's likely you've exhausted a long list of healing options just as I did, yet you still feel stuck. The good news is, *you're reading this book*—a book that will help you finally discover the innate tools for self-healing that your body has naturally carried all along. As I type this, I can hear the collective cry from so many of my clients during the years: "After decades of suffering, I wish I had known about these practices sooner!" At last, my friend, you're on the precipice of true and lasting healing. I'm beyond excited for you.

In this moment, I'm brought back to the present with my daughter. She gently sleeps with a dreamy grin spread across her face. As I observe her, I see me. And again, I'm reminded of younger Britt. Had you told her that she'd one day write a book, filled with personal tales of hope, healing, and a tried-and-true roadmap for recovery, she wouldn't have believed you. The truth is, throughout a good majority of my time on this Earth, my brain *lovingly* suppressed many of the memories I gathered to share with you in this book. I'd liken crafting these pages to rummaging through a dust-covered attic filled with keepsakes, portraits, and boxes sealed for decades. Each box packed with experiences, both good and bad, that had been tucked away and hidden out of sight.

You, too, have an attic to explore, filled with a spectrum of experiences—joy, grief, love, fear, and more. As I slowly sift through my stories in this book, I hope the learned tools and my own therapeutic process provide you comfort and courage to do just the same. *Body-First Healing* will empower you with my proven framework to healing that has compassionately guided thousands of clients globally and removed the defensive walls that were keeping them stuck, allowing them to re-create a life deeply centered around presence, connection, vitality, and joy. Whatever pain has led you to this point, I hope you know there's more to life than just surviving.

Now let's rediscover who you are, before the pain and armor told you who to be.

Lovingly,
Britt

PART I

How and Why Trauma Lives in the Body

Introducing Resourcing

As you journey into the pages of this book, you might find that the stories or concepts shared may trigger feelings of unease within you. This is only natural when reflecting on the nature of trauma and how it shows up in your life today. To support your capacity to move through that unease, I'd like to introduce you to a foundational element of Somatic Experiencing, known as "resourcing."

A resource is any experience that cultivates more settling, stability, or calm in your body or nervous system; more presence, more spaciousness, more breath. It is the first step for creating a deeper capacity for nervous system regulation, and it is necessary for moving through stress. It's important to create a foundation or "toolbox" of resources of anything that brings with it a feeling or sense of okayness, goodness, or slight betterness.

These resources can be internal (such as a pleasant emotion, sensation, visualization, or memory) or external (such as a slow orientation or observation of the space around you with your senses, co-regulation or connection with another, or supportive movement).

As you navigate through this book, I encourage you to lean into the resources that support you as needed. You can find much more detail about resourcing, including step-by-step instructions and some go-to practices, in chapter 16.

CHAPTER 1

Healing with a Body-First Approach

I've spent most of my thirty-six years of life trying to piece together the tarnished puzzle of my traumatic younger years. I have little memory of it all; I've only heard whispered tales passed down by family members comfortable enough to share. And so, I've become an expert investigator into my own background. Although I don't remember much of my upbringing, I remember vividly how I *felt*— unstable, insecure, afraid, and disconnected. As I turned the corner into adulthood with these same feelings in tow, I began to realize that this sense of being "unlovable" wasn't normal or healthy. That began my relentless journey to uncover: Who was younger Britt? And what experiences and events made her who she is today?

Throughout this book, I'll share and compassionately explore what I discovered and the nuances of my story. But for now, I'll give you a rough sketch of my experiences growing up and how I can now see they shaped me.

The Concrete Bottom

I was born in 1988, at Sharp Grossmont Hospital in Southern California. What should have been a beautifully memorable day was seemingly anything but. Right after my birth, I was taken from my mother and placed into foster care because methamphetamine was found in my system. And my father? He had no intention of being a part of my life. Although I would eventually be reunited with my mom, the internal damage was done: The seeds of unworthiness and fear of abandonment were planted into my developing subconscious. In my younger years I was insecure and disconnected from myself, and this began my patterns of codependency and my tendency to appease others so that I would be accepted.

Years later, this abandonment wound was exacerbated by the sudden loss of my brother in a car accident when we were teenagers. Spiraling out of control and desperate to numb my unbearable feelings, I soon became a slave to alcohol and drugs. However, in my attempt to run from the grief, my self-medicating nearly ran me into my own grave. I ended up in a hospital, where I flatlined from alcohol poisoning. Determined to live, I began attending Alcoholics Anonymous, because surely the problem was the alcohol—or so I was told by my therapist.

Two years later, at the age of twenty, I was brutally raped and beaten by a stranger who had helped me change a flat tire. Even though I assisted in putting this man behind bars for sixty years, the very public and very painful two-year trial process left me even more traumatized. I once again retreated to my old patterns of wanting to numb my suffering by continuing to drink so much that *I* ended up in a jail cell after a violent drunken night out, not even thirty days after the trial sentencing. (We'll get to those details later.) This time, full of rage and despair, I officially became a version of myself I didn't recognize.

As is often said, you have to hit rock bottom before you can start to make the changes you know you need to make. In my case, *my bottom was the cold, hard concrete of a six-by-eight-foot jail cell.*

It was there that I was forced to sit with the discomfort of all that I had been avoiding for so many years. No pills, no alcohol, no chaos, and no dysfunction to distract me; it was just me and my feelings, alone together in a cage. I felt like a pressure cooker ready to explode. The anger, the grief, the shame, the fear—they came crashing into that bare cell in intense waves of sensation and emotion. I found myself shaking, trembling, crying, sweating, wailing, and moaning. I didn't learn until later that this was my body releasing—or "discharging"— the stuck and stored survival energy (adrenaline) from the past. I was surprised to make it out alive, but I did. And amazingly enough, I felt lighter and remarkably better.

During those few days, the release and processing of decades-old pain gave way to a profound clarity I hadn't ever experienced. In those crystal-clear moments of reflection, it wasn't lost on me that I was behind bars at the same time as my perpetrator. This enlightenment revealed that he and I perhaps had more in common than I'd initially realized. During the trial, his defense team had highlighted his trau-matic upbringing: He was raised by an aunt as one of fifteen kids, and he'd had poor schooling, as well as mental and physical health issues. We both were dealt an ugly hand in life, and we both were offered the same choice: Allow your pain to make you better, or allow it to make you bitter. He made his choice, and he'd spend the next sixty years be-hind bars, being reminded of his decision. And me? I was seemingly venturing down the same path. At a crossroads, I had to decide if this was truly how my life would go.

When I went to court after three days in jail, I faced a judge who knew me from my sexual assault case. The words she spoke to me were profound and have stuck with me: "We're going to drop the charges, but . . ." she paused and repeated, "but, you need to learn to *live with your pain* better."

Those four words—*live with your pain*. That was it, the turning point when everything just clicked. She didn't say to get over the pain, or get past it and *start over*. She said to live *with* the pain.

I realized in that moment that I couldn't run anymore, and that the path of numbing, avoiding, and "least resistance" was actually proving to be more destructive than the alternative of facing the pain of the past. It was time to surrender and remove the decades of armor I had built up. Only then could I find from within the self-compassion and resilience to receive the healing I so rightfully deserved.

The Body: The Missing Puzzle Piece

Until that point, I had spent most of my recovery sitting behind closed doors across from conventional, buttoned-up therapists who insisted I verbally recall and replay each excruciating moment of my twenty-plus years of severe trauma. "Exposure-based therapy," they called it. We revisited and rehashed each event, as best as I could remember. We talked and talked ad nauseum, always staying strictly in the fast lane of thought, story, cognition, and meaning and rarely slowing down enough to allow emotions to emerge. Meanwhile, my body felt like a buried explosive, a charge just waiting to be detonated by the tiniest trigger or movement from above. If I expressed discomfort or difficult emotions, my therapists would rush to encourage me to think about "something positive." Yet, the explosive was still there.

Despite the therapists' best intentions, I'd leave these sessions feeling more guarded, anxious, and hopeless than before. The more I *talked*, the more stuck I became. Given no tools to process and manage the overwhelming discomfort of my body—rage, grief, fear, constriction, and dissociation, to name a few—the only temporary fix was to rely on the cocktail of medications I'd been prescribed for my many diagnoses: attention deficit hyperactivity disorder (ADHD), anxiety, depression, post-traumatic stress disorder (PTSD), and more. It was a vicious cycle, and I began to doubt not only the medical system, but also myself. I knew that something had to change.

Still reeling from the profound healing experience I'd had in that jail cell, I decided to take my recovery into my own hands, and I set out on a quest to understand the imprint my traumas had left. Through this journey, I began to discover groundbreaking evidence, not talked about in mainstream recovery circles, that healing begins when you get out of your head, out of the story, and into your body. For me, learning this concept was revolutionary: *Wait, so healing doesn't have to do with* talking? *It has to do with* feeling? Drawing from the decades-old science, I focused on three important concepts:

- Trauma can easily be described as any experience that's too overwhelming for the nervous system to cope with. After trauma, our nervous system can become locked in states of protection (fight, flight, shutdown, freeze, or fawn), further wreaking havoc on our lives, relationships, and health.

- The nervous system doesn't operate through thoughts, words, or cognition, but rather through the somatic (body-oriented) experience of feelings, sensations, and emotions—a language never truly explored in conventional therapy.

- Humans are considered "bottom-up" beings, because 80 percent of the messages sent through our vagus nerve (our information superhighway) are from the body to the brain, and only 20 percent are from the brain to the body. Bottom line: Your body has a lot more say when it comes to how you show up in your life and in the world. This is why I couldn't just talk through it or create a "positive mindset" to find my way out of the anxiety, depression, and grief. I had to *feel* my way out.

In summary, I discovered that trauma isn't created by the event; it comes from the nervous system's impulse to subconsciously repeat, in the present, the responses it enlisted to survive the past. Some people stuck in this cycle shrink (shutdown) or run away (flight or flee) when conflict presents itself. Others appease (fawn) and sacrifice their own desires or boundaries to be accepted. Some blow up (fight) when things feel out of their control. Many of us experience more than one of these responses, and our lives become ruled by them. Consider these as survival or management strategies that have overstayed their welcome.

During my research, I took a deep dive into Peter Levine's work, which introduced me to the world of somatic or body-oriented healing. In the 1970s, Levine made groundbreaking observations of animals in the wild, which led him to ask an intriguing question: Why are animals in the wild, although threatened routinely, rarely traumatized?

Levine discovered that when faced with threat, wild animals employ instinctual impulses through their body (like shaking, trembling, growling, playing dead, etc.) that allow them to process, neutralize, and release the high level of survival energy (adrenaline) that is associated with the nervous system's threat response cycle. His research concluded that although humans possess nervous system responses *virtually identical to those in animals* (thanks to our shared mammalian and reptilian brain structures, which we'll explore in detail later), these instinctual impulses are often interrupted or *overridden* by our neocortex or human brain—our "rational mind."

THE ORIGINS OF SOMATIC EXPERIENCING

It should come as no surprise that Somatic Experiencing, a revolutionary trauma recovery method previously considered "fringe," was born in the 1970s in Berkeley, California—the epicenter of progressive mindsets and intellectual curiosity at the time. Berkeley's worldwide reputation as being an imaginative center of academic freedom made it the perfect place for Dr. Peter Levine to begin his research on the effects of trauma on both the body and the mind. With doctorates in biophysics from the University of California,

Berkeley, and psychology from International University, Los Angeles, Levine was driven by his personal adversity, his private work with trauma survivors, and his observations of animals recovering in the wild. His studies led him to the conclusion that talk therapy as a method to resolve trauma has limitations, because it doesn't effectively address the accumulated arousal (stress hormones) that is entrenched and stuck within the body and nervous system.

Levine's observation that wild animals can "shake it off" led him to ask why *human* animals get stuck in their trauma and wild animals do not. His remarkable research created the basis for today's Somatic Experiencing. As he wrote in *Healing Trauma: A Pioneering Program for Restoring the Wisdom of Your Body*: "A threatened human being must discharge all the energy mobilized to negotiate the threat or it becomes a victim of trauma. This residual energy does not simply go away. It persists in the body and often forces the formation of a wide variety of symptoms, e.g. anxiety, depression, and psychosomatic and behavioral problems. These symptoms are the organism's (body's) way of containing the undischarged residual energy."

Levine leaned into his findings in nature and paired his theoretical approach with the hard science of the Polyvagal Theory, which was developed by his close friend and colleague, Stephen Porges. In the 1990s, Levine and Porges finally put body psychotherapy on the map. Today, Levine's pioneering Somatic Experiencing method of body-centered trauma resolution has been taught and embraced by more than 60,000 practitioners in more than 45 countries. His visionary work is celebrated all around the globe, and he has received some of the highest accolades from the most prestigious international medical institutions and organizations, including the Psychotherapy Networker Lifetime Achievement Award in 2020. Levine heartwarmingly reflected on the award in an article published by the *International Body Psychotherapy Journal*: "Getting this award, not from a body-centered field, but from very traditional talk therapy representatives, made it clear to me that the genie was out of the box; that it was no longer a fringe movement. Embodied psychotherapy is now part of the mainstream. Because again, what I discovered in the late 60's and early 70's was that trauma is something that not only affects the brain . . . it primarily affects the body."[1]

In essence, when these stuck survival hormones are interrupted, either by an overwhelming circumstance or our own doing, they create chronic mental and physical health conditions within the brain and the body. One thing that compounds the problem for humans is that we are the only species on the planet with a split mind of conscious and subconscious experiences. As a result, we can often "get in our head" (or, in other words, our conscious mind) by over-conceptualizing our feelings, rather than just allowing ourselves to feel and process those feelings so the accompanying survival energy, or adrenaline, tied to them can then be *experienced, expressed,* and *expelled*. As we often say in the somatic space, over-thinking is an under-feeling problem. Here are some examples of how that can play out in our lives: We minimize or suppress our frustration or anger (fight response) to "keep the peace" or "be a nice boy or girl," we push away or override our fear or anxiety for the sake of "being calm," we hold back our tears and "suck it up" or "stay positive," we scroll and distract to escape what doesn't feel good.

The body-centered understanding made so much sense to me: Feel it to heal it. It was no wonder recall therapy had little to no effect on me. Although I felt grateful for my body's innate ability to quite literally keep me alive and protected throughout all the traumatic seasons of my life, I was done being stuck in survival mode.

It was in my season of research and discovery that I made the choice to switch to a body-first or somatic approach to healing. It didn't take long after doing so for the laundry list of symptoms therapists had attributed to my "diagnoses"—the crippling panic attacks, the suicidal ideation, the eating disorders, the ADHD, the fog of depression, the impulse to self-medicate, and even the attraction I had to codependent and abusive relationships—to magically lift and disappear. Within months, I threw away my pills. By coming back into my body and its natural wisdom, and finally welcoming hard feelings, I was healed in remarkable ways, and I rediscovered who I *actually was*—before the pain and the armor told me who to be.

Now, more than a decade later, as a Somatic Experiencing Practitioner (SEP™) and trauma educator, I've made this work my life's mission and have guided thousands of trauma survivors worldwide to the path of recovery.

A Trauma-Informed World

Before venturing into the Body-First Healing Roadmap, it's important that we first take a peek behind the curtain so we can better understand how we've created the culture of *survival and stuckness* that we are currently living in.

The rise of chronic physical and mental illness can easily be attributed to one thing: we created a world our nervous system doesn't want to live in. Think of it this way: your nervous system is the security camera of your life, always operating in the subconscious, the background, to protect you from anything it perceives to not be safe. When perceived danger is near, it goes into active states of survival: fight, flight, shutdown, freeze, or fawn. At the same time, stress (aka survival) hormones are released at high amounts throughout the body to prepare us for battle. As survival becomes priority number one, all other working systems of the brain and body (immune, digestion, musculoskeletal, hormone) fall to the back burner so that the nervous system can do its job well.

When faced with prolonged exposure to "perceived threat," the nervous system can become chronically stuck in these states of survival—wreaking havoc on our physical and mental health, which further creates higher levels of stress hormones in the body and brain. It's a vicious cycle to get out of. And one that many of us face today, in our modern world. Here are some of the threats we face that contribute to this state of survival and stuckness:

- The societal pressure to do more, make more, "succeed more" to the point of burnout

- The divisive political climates we live in

- The fear of volatile economies

- The judgment faced when we express emotion or share vulnerability

- The environmental toxins our bodies are exposed to (in food, air, water, etc.)

- The constant bombardment and exposure to catastrophic news and world events

- The harsh guilt we face when we set boundaries and prioritize ourselves

- The reliance on technology that keeps us blissfully disconnected from ourselves and the present

There's perceived threat at every corner, yet we wonder why we're so sick. So how do we get unstuck from these survival states? The Body-First Healing Roadmap will guide you through that profound process, but for now, here are some simple steps:

Step 1: Slow down.

Step 2: Get in your body.

Step 3: Get present.

Step 4: Validate what sucks and what's hard, AND soak in what's good (we call these "glimmers").

Step 5: Give more power to what you can actually control and sway.

Step 6: Find your regulating resources: nature, connection with others, movement, expression, play, and more.

The goal in all of this isn't to make the threat disappear, because that's truly impossible, especially in our world today. The goal is to find ways to blossom in the mess, to regulate in the chaos, to find safety—despite the danger.

~~What's Wrong With Them?~~ What Happened to Them?

Shortly after I woke, there was a doctor standing at the end of my bed. "Brittany, you're in the hospital. You arrived here last night by ambulance with alcohol poisoning and a Blood Alcohol Content of .38. To be frank, it's a miracle you're alive."

Let's rewind. In 2007 I moved from the Midwest to New York City to start my freshman year of college. I had received a Division I athletic scholarship to play lacrosse. On paper and on the outside, I seemed to have it all together. Yet behind the mask was a struggling young girl, who hid from her new team and friends the grief of losing her brother, her best friend, just three years prior in a car accident.

Desperate to start over in a new place, I no longer wanted to be treated with pity, tiptoed around, and seen as "the girl who's grieving." So I drank the pain away and kept it hidden. Yet in the shadows, the sadness grew stronger and became more unbearable and impossible to ignore. With the rise of pain came an increase of my self-medicating, until eventually it gave way to self-destruction, nearly taking my life on that fateful night.

What's ingrained in my mind seventeen years later isn't the horror of waking up in that hospital bed, but the torturous response of my coaches and community that followed in the aftermath. I can vividly recall sitting in my coach's office, a windowless room in the basement of our athletic center. I can still feel the rage and disdain that my coach and assistant coach spewed at me. I remember her screaming in my face; she was so close that I can still feel the hot breath and the spit landing on my cheek. The curse words and name-calling.

I walked away from that meeting fully internalizing every word: I was a disgrace to our team. I had tarnished our reputation of having the highest GPA in the country, being honored with the distinction of "Division I Merit Status." I was a stain on our prestigious school. I learned that our status as a team was more important than my individual well-being. Recovery came secondary to public image. It didn't matter that I was grieving, it didn't matter that I was living in unbearable turmoil and pain. "We all have a past, get over it!" was the only recognition my trauma received.

I received the message loud and clear that I was no longer wanted on the team. It took only a week for my coaches to begin their campaign to ostracize me, turn my teammates against me, punish me, and push me out. I could handle the daily hour-long sprints before the sun came up each morning as punishment. But what broke me was the daily hour-long sprints that my entire team was forced to do while I sat on the bleachers watching. Sprint sessions so intense that a trash can was put at the end line for my teammates to get sick in. Sprints so intense that with every whistle my body flinched, and tears fell as my teammates, who I once leaned on for friendship and support, now glared at me with hatred and rejection.

When all was said and done, I was gone from the school by November with nothing but broken friendships and broken memories in the rearview. Five years later, I found myself standing on a stage in front of a collegiate audience, sharing about my life, my journey to healing, and challenging misconceptions and attitudes surrounding recovery and trauma. Most important, I shared about how we can all contribute to a more trauma-informed world. One where we no longer look at people's pain as a burden. Where we no longer ask "What's wrong with them?" and instead get curious about "What happened to them?" Where we put well-being in front of image. Looking back, I wish eighteen-year-old Britt would've known all that would come from her pain and adversity.

An Era of Disconnection

This book comes at a pivotal time in our world. We've Jedi mind-tricked our way into becoming masters of emotional avoidance, allowing us to deny the invisible wounds that haunt us and keep us stuck. We've replaced *feeling* with conceptualizing, overriding discomfort or difficult emotions with well-intentioned practices of mindfulness, meditation, and toxic positivity. We've glorified a destructive culture of *emotional suppression*, in which we unknowingly subscribe to anything that keeps us blissfully distracted and disconnected from our bodies, such as our addiction to working endless hours and scrolling mindlessly on our phones. Even our efforts at combatting mental health issues ignore the mind-body connection and the implicit wisdom that the body holds over the brain.

Bottom line: We're in trouble. Through social media, we have immediate access to intimate and often grotesque details of the pain of the world in a way that's never been experienced in human history. Our brains and bodies aren't yet equipped or haven't yet been given the tools to help us live with the exposure and emotional impact of this suffering.

In particular, our younger generations are struggling at unprecedented rates. More and more kids are being diagnosed with ADHD, depression, and anxiety than ever before. Gen Z (those born between 1997 and 2012) was even deemed by the Centers for Disease Control and Prevention (CDC) as the "loneliest generation" in our history.[2] We look at these statistics and ask, "What's wrong with that generation?" without considering the environment around them—they are living in a world full of *disconnection*, from ourselves, others, and the world. It's like a fish that is sick because its fishbowl isn't clean. The addictions and diseases our children are suffering from are merely a *natural response* to an unnatural environment, one that worships the mind while discarding the ancient and primal intellect of the body.

And then, along came COVID-19. Until the pandemic hit, most of us had become experts at suppressing or bulldozing our way through discomfort. Although it brought trauma, too, the pandemic gave us a rare opportunity to finally sit in isolation and quarantine with the traumas we had been running from, much like my experience in the jail cell. In isolation, we couldn't suppress or distract in ways we once might have—staying late at work, socializing, or drinking away our painful reality. We couldn't be consumed by the chaos of dysfunctional relationships. We found more support online, where the message was that it's "okay to not be okay." There was a collective realization that our world was hurting, and a greater understanding that every one of us is carrying around invisible wounds.

I welcomed this shift in perspective. I distinctly remember a conversation I had with a speaking colleague in 2016. As we chatted over coffee, I shared with her that I wanted to talk more publicly about the topic of trauma. Her response? "That'd be career suicide. Trauma isn't a *sexy* topic. People just aren't ready for that."

At the time, she may have been right. Trauma was thought to be "too much" or "too heavy" for the masses, who didn't have the capacity, or patience, to digest the realities of it all. But during COVID, a cultural moment of global healing began to take place. The shift was one that I had long advocated for—I hoped we could upend conventional thinking and move to a more enlightened and natural approach to healing trauma.

I can say with confidence that we are now experiencing a global healing movement. In my practice, I have seen more patients filling the virtual and in-person waiting rooms of our therapists and practitioners than ever before. Social media platforms like Instagram and TikTok have become the newest community forum for multifaceted explorations of trauma recovery. The few books published on healing trauma through the body, such as *The Body Keeps the Score: Brain, Mind, and Body in the Healing of Trauma* by Bessel van der Kolk (first published in 2014), finally hit the bestseller list. The paradigm of modern therapy is transforming right before our eyes, and fast.

Healing with a Body-First Approach

The old debate used to be that trauma wasn't "sexy enough," but now trauma is almost "*too* sexy," or "too trendy." In fact, a 2022 study noted that the term *trauma* appeared in psychology journal articles in the 2010s at a rate almost twenty times higher than it did in the 1970s. This magnifying lens led to the rise of trauma recovery books written by researchers, doctors, and psychology experts in the field. They're educational and informative, but most are more like textbooks, and they stick to the now-outdated standard of care: talk therapy, prescription medications, and symptom management.

The biggest limitation of the recall or exposure-based therapeutic model (which I'll discuss in more detail in the next chapter) is that most medical professionals assume that trauma is about the event itself. They believe healing necessitates a deep dive into what happened, by remembering and rehashing all the difficult details. However, research shows that exposure therapy, a form of desensitization therapy, can actually worsen our symptoms and further overwhelm our nervous system—pushing us into a physiological freeze or shutdown response.[3] This state is only activated when the nervous system is so unbelievably overwhelmed and has exhausted all other options. It's our "life-or-death" state, where we numb ourselves to pain. Yet numbing is not the same thing as healing. And although externally we may appear to be "better" (less anxious or angry, for instance), internally there's still a sea of survival hormones that needs to be experienced, expressed, and expelled.

The word *desensitization* means "moving away from or out of sensitization or sensation." *Yet sensation is the first language of the nervous system and crucially needed in the exploration and facilitation of healing.* As Peter Levine says, "Trauma isn't found in the event; it's found in the nervous system."

This is why many of my clients come to me after years of being stuck in survival mode. Despite their best efforts to heal, they're still left with the debilitating symptoms that accompany their stuckness. They've become all too familiar with the never-ending and often codependent hamster wheel of exhausting therapy appointments, prescriptions, and merely *getting by*. One of my clients even told me that, after therapy, she'd head right for the local bar because she was so anxious and agitated and re-traumatized by having to consistently recall her trauma. That was me as well. Even with years of therapy alongside many well-meaning mental health professionals, I was still drinking to numb myself and making destructive life choices. Like many of the clients who I've supported, talking about my trauma was not the key to my healing. It was the *lock*.

What's the alternative? Effective and lasting healing begins in the body. As world-renowned trauma expert Dr. Gabor Maté puts it, "Trauma is not what happens *to* you (i.e., the event), trauma is what happens *inside of* you, as a result of what happened to you." Because trauma is *first* experienced and stored in the body, it should be healed there first.

As more studies are being done, the decades-old science behind somatic healing is finally starting to emerge in the mainstream. Take it from one of my former somatic clients: "As a former licensed therapist, I'd love to say that while I adore my profession and have indeed helped a lot of people, talk therapy does *not* work as it should when dealing with trauma. It wasn't until I understood my nervous system and worked toward regulation that I got my life back!"

HANNAH'S STORY

I spent my childhood and early twenties being diagnosed with a variety of mental illnesses and chronic diseases, all while being in weekly talk therapy that was getting me nowhere. I had become a mom in my early twenties, and my physical and mental health were only getting worse. I was trying new medications monthly without any success and, sadly, just living a very painful life, both mentally and physically. I was stuck. Fortunately, a friend suggested that I work on my nervous system to help me heal. I had never thought about my nervous system or really knew anything about it. I began researching online for information about the nervous system and its ties to chronic disease and overall health. Brittany's name came up right away. And as soon as I started watching her videos, I just *knew*—I had a gut feeling that this was what would finally help me both in my mental and emotional struggles but also in my chronic illnesses. I'd spent most of my life in talk therapy but was at the point that I was talking in circles, never feeling like things were changing or shifting for me, and when I would leave my sessions, I would feel worse.

I began the course, Body-First Healing Program (BFHP), and am grateful to have been a one-on-one client of Brittany's ever since. I benefited more from the BFHP in a few short months than I had my entire life in talk therapy. I had been diagnosed with multiple mental illnesses, but what I actually had was a dysregulated nervous system and a lot of complex developmental trauma I needed to unravel. I finally felt like the power was in my hands to take ownership of what was going on in my body, and it wasn't just some mental illness I had no control of. Immediately after learning the science behind the nervous system, I was able to shift my entire thinking about my mental and physical ailments.

Somatically, during the last two years, Brittany has guided me and my nervous system on the path to healing. With her help, I've been able to work through a lot of things in my life and childhood that I didn't even realize were affecting me and creating physical ailments, too—chronic pain, headaches, and stomach issues. Bringing clarity to my emotions, and learning how my body has held onto everything I've ever experienced but never allowed my body to feel, has been life-changing. I am on a journey to bring more and more awareness to my body and to understand specifically *where* in my body I feel my emotions and experiences. I have begun to break free of this physical and mental pain while bringing my mind and body to a place of ease and regulation. I am building my capacity to walk through life with a strong and well-versed nervous system.

I feel so grateful to have stumbled across Brittany's information online when I did, as I know her knowledge, teachings, and passion for the nervous system will be incredibly monumental in so many lives, just as they have been in mine. I'm so thankful to have escaped the system that never helped me. Instead, *I was able to look within my own body to find healing.* This work is so important, and I will be passing it on to my children in every way I can so they don't have to grow up experiencing life the way I did for so many years.

Introducing Somatic Experiencing®—the Basics

Let's start with the basics: The goal of Somatic Experiencing is to better help you *be with the experience of your body, such as sensations and emotions,* rather than avoiding or suppressing. We aim to make room for our emotions, not remove them. Why is this important? Let's first consider the commonly used phrase "emotionally charged." Did you know that your emotions do, in fact, carry an energetic charge?

When your nervous system perceives threat, it armors up to protect you through the initiation of the threat response cycle. This physiological response aims to provide immediate protection through the release of the mobilizing or "charged" stress hormones adrenaline and cortisol, engaging your body's natural impulse to fight, flight, shut down, freeze, or fawn. Survival mode is great for the short term but it's not meant to be lived in, nor is our body designed to withstand it over long periods. Further, when we ignore or suppress that charge (i.e., emotional avoidance), it stays stuck within the body. Think of it like this: When we bury our emotions or our trauma, we bury it *alive*—creating an internal environment that's fueled by toxic stress hormones and more vulnerable to chronic conditions.

A four-step sequence of physiological reactions occur during a healthy stress or threat response cycle:

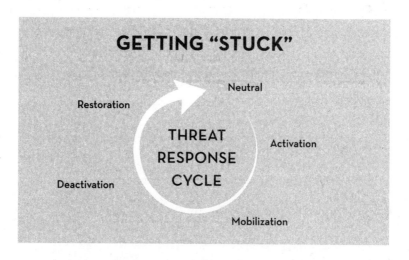

1. **Neutral:** You're in your "safe and connected state," where you feel secure, present, and at ease.

2. **Activation:** A perceived threat triggers your nervous system to go into a survival response of either fight, flight, shutdown, freeze, or fawn. The stress hormones adrenaline and cortisol are released into the body.

3. **Mobilization:** If you can successfully allow the natural impulse of your nervous system to complete, then you are able to release, aka "discharge," the survival hormones from your body.

4. **Deactivation:** Following a discharge comes a natural "deactivation," when your system comes back into restoration, ease, and then returns to neutral.

From a simpler approach, we can consider it in terms of what I call the *4 E's of Emotion*:

1. **Emerge:** A feeling emerges in the body (example: anxiety).

2. **Experience:** We allow the feeling to be felt and experienced, observing the emotions and sensations present (example: constriction in the chest, increased heart rate, heat in the limbs, trembling).

3. **Express:** A natural impulse or expression may follow as we make room for the somatic experience (example: voicing a boundary, leaving or escaping, crying, laughing, shaking).

4. **Expel:** As we express, the body naturally releases or discharges the emotional charge of stress hormones.

Let's explore an example of the threat response cycle in everyday life: You're driving, singing along to your favorite song, feeling present and at ease (step 1—neutral). You suddenly hear sirens and realize flashing lights are coming up quickly behind you. You look down at the dashboard. You're speeding. Panic and anxiety set in as the possibility that you could get pulled over hits you. You quickly shut off the music and grip both hands on the wheel. You're now sweating, you feel heat, your heart's racing, and your eyes narrowly focus on the rearview mirror (step 2—activation). You start to make your way to the shoulder as the car slows down. Now on the side of the road, you hold your breath as the police car flies past you. You let out a loud and relieving "AGHHH, THANK GOD!" followed by a brief moment to literally shake it off through your hands and limbs. You might even laugh and let out an audible "Whew." The movement and vocalization allow the adrenaline from the anxiety to be experienced, expressed, and expelled (step 3—mobilization). You take a few deep breaths. After you've oriented back to the present moment, you creep back onto the road and slowly return to a state of ease—heart slowing, body temperature cooling, relaxed muscles, and music back on (step 4—deactivation).

This is a beautiful example of your nervous system's *natural ability* to go back and forth—what we call "pendulate"—between activation (triggered) and deactivation (not triggered). (We will talk more about pendulation in part II.) One way we can interrupt this cycle is when we don't allow ourselves to feel or express. The other way is when the experience is something that either feels like too much, too soon, or too fast, and our nervous system becomes overwhelmed. Both scenarios cause us to get stuck in the activation and mobilization stages.

This was the case for me, after I was assaulted in 2009 by a stranger who helped me change a flat tire. During the experience, my nervous system tried to mobilize and fight back to protect myself, but my perpetrator was able to overpower me. This caused the survival charge to remain stored in my body and physiology and keep me stuck in an activated state of fight. Following the assault, I became angry, resentful, and full of rage—qualities that were in direct opposition to my usual gentle nature. I became someone I didn't recognize.

It all took a turn in 2011, when, a few weeks after my perpetrator's sentencing hearing, I was out drinking with someone who was also drinking and driving, too. (I always say this was a good indication of being at one of my lowest points in life.) After he was pulled over and arrested, the police officers tried to pull me out of the passenger seat to give me a ride home. However, in my impaired state, I had a flash-back of the night of my assault, of a strange man touching me in a car. I snapped, as my nervous system violently went into a trauma re-enactment to fight back, desperate to complete the threat response cycle that was incomplete from the initial assault. That's how I ended up in a jail cell.

My story illustrates that when our nervous system gets trapped in a survival, protective state, our personality can change. Five distinct personality types are given rise by our trauma response. I call them "stuck personality types." We will explore them in great length in the rest of the book, but for now, here is a short description:

1. **Fight:** The angry one
2. **Flight:** The overachiever or anxious worrier
3. **Shutdown:** The "lazy" introvert
4. **Functional freeze:** The one who "muscles through"
5. **Fawn:** The people-pleaser

In the season of life following my assault, I got stuck in the "fight" response/personality type. But other people may respond differently. By using a body-first approach to heal the nervous system and release the chronic stress energy that has become stuck and stored in the body, we can easily come back to the restored, regulated, and authentic versions of ourselves.

Slow, Gentle, and Present Self-Healing

Somatic Experiencing isn't fixated on the past. It focuses more on how a traumatic event or experience is impacting you today, in the *present*. Remember, trauma isn't found in the event, but in the survival responses of the nervous system.

Now, this doesn't mean that we minimize or avoid pain, because we know that avoiding isn't the same thing as healing. Instead, we equip you with somatic tools and practices to welcome in and process the discomfort in a tolerable way. We validate and create a greater capacity within your nervous system to be with anger, fear, shame, anxiety, etc.—just like that judge encouraged me to do. We're ultimately aiding your nervous system in becoming more resilient, which will help you not just to heal, but also to better manage stress and challenges in your everyday life.

So how do we find regulation in the nervous system? We employ a "safety-first" approach by starting with a foundation of feeling "resourced," or safe in your body. We do this by building more things that feel good—your resources—into your daily life and routine so your nervous system has tools to fall back on when healing and life in general feel too hard. When you're back at baseline, you can then slowly start processing the actual trauma.

It's also important to highlight that it's not about feeling safe all the time. Because the reality is, it's impossible to feel safe all the time—whether that unsafety is real or perceived—such as when someone judges us, an experience feels out of our control, or our trust has been broken. Feeling unsafe is not just normal in the face of day-to-day obstacles, but it's also expected. It's a fact of life. So instead of attempting to feel safe 24/7, we aim to create a deeper ability to feel and move through the sensations of unsafety when they do inevitably arise.

As you'll see in part II, once learned, these gentle somatic practices can be done on your own. It's true: you get to harness your innate tools from within so you can *self-heal* in the ways your body was built to. These are small and convenient practices, easily woven into your everyday life, that can give you profound relief. And over time, the cumulative effect will create greater resilience in your nervous system's natural ability to move through activation.

Within Somatic Experiencing, you take small and tolerable steps toward healing, or what we Somatic Experiencing Practitioners call "titration." Just as you'd titrate slowly off a medication you've been on for a long time to minimize harmful side effects, titration gives your nervous system a chance to slowly catch up to the present and regulate (or get unstuck), without overwhelming it further or exacerbating your symptoms. The goal is to stretch you without stressing you—we take off one piece of protective armor at a time, which in turn creates *sustainable* healing. No Band-Aid approaches here.

The Body-First Healing Roadmap follows a path of titration as well, with the beginning chapters of this book easing you into the knowledge and scientific framework of the modalities we'll explore, the middle chapters preparing you with the tools to do the work, and the final sections guiding you deep into the actual application of somatic healing. This slow and safe method is exactly why some clients get to the end of this work amazed that their life has completely transformed, yet they'll swear it never felt like too much.

Somatic Experiencing proves that treating trauma does not mean you have to be curled up in a ball in your therapist's office, sobbing in agonizing pain as you are told to relive your traumatic situation over and over to "get over it." It is quite the opposite—it is gentle and should never be overwhelming.

Somatic healing saved my life—a life I thought I'd never get back. It returned me to the wholeness of who I was. It gave me hope, compassionate understanding, and tools to face whatever lies ahead. I'm honored to guide you in this work, with the full belief it will do the same for you.

CHAPTER 2

The Top-Down and Bottom-Up Approaches for Trauma

W hen I reflect on my younger years, I can report with confidence that I was a pretty average student, with a GPA range right between a C+ and a B—. I never really loved school, or at least the learning or reading parts of it. Sports and socializing were where I excelled. And it made sense, really. When your nervous system is chronically stuck in survival (fighting, fleeing, or hiding from the imaginary lion from the past), the brain isn't really primed for learning. In fact, when the amygdala (survival brain) takes over, the prefrontal cortex (thinking/learning brain) becomes inhibited.

This explained a lot. Like why I was always spaced out in class, pulled into a perpetual state of distraction, daydreaming, and dissociating. Words often blurred on pages, causing me to have to reread paragraphs and entire chapters over and over to get the information to stick. Most of the time that didn't work so I became an expert cheater instead. My brain fog was so bad that I sometimes wondered if I had a learning disability, like my older brother did. It turns out, there was never anything wrong with me, and likely never anything wrong with my brother either. My brain was simply prioritizing survival. In fact, I'd later come to find that when my brain and body weren't stuck in survival mode, I actually *loved* learning.

In particular, I discovered that I loved learning about trauma and the science behind it. I loved it so much that I eventually became a trauma educator myself, leading forensic neurobiology trauma trainings for private and government organizations worldwide—which in hindsight is pretty remarkable, given my previously mediocre school performance. In my wildest classroom daydreams, high-school Britt never would have imagined that she'd one day be expertly educating our nation's military, the Department of Justice, investigative violent crime units, international crisis centers, students and administrators in higher education, and more about the intricate details of trauma: how it resides within us and how we can heal. Yet here we are.

This is where our roadmap begins, with the science that gifts us evidence and self-awareness that the ways we behave, think, and feel make *perfect sense* through a trauma-informed lens of self-protection, not self-sabotage. The science proves to us, once again, that we are not broken and do not need fixing. And it's this self-awareness that fosters compassion, acceptance, and even gratitude for the armor we've had to bear. Over time, it takes the place of the self-inflicting judgment, shame, and confusion we've carried about why we are the way we are. Knowledge, or context, is truly powerful in the pursuit of healing.

The Whole Pie

I like to view healing in general as one big pie, with a handful of different slices, or modalities. Everyone's pie is made of different slices, because what works for one person doesn't always work for another. Talk therapy is one slice of the pie, Somatic Experiencing is another slice, Internal Family Systems (IFS) is a slice, neurofeedback is a slice, EMDR another, and so on. One isn't better than the other, and in fact, most healing modalities are incredibly effective when utilized at the right time, in the right way, for the right person. What I'm attempting to say is, there's space for all of it.

I also want to clarify that I will never claim that conventional talk therapy is bad or useless for healing trauma. On the contrary. Cognition, understanding, and narrative reframing are *incredibly important* aspects when it comes to recovery—as long as the meaning-making doesn't ignore what the body is also trying to convey. Unfortunately, when it comes to trauma recovery, mainstream medicine has pigeonholed us into one modality.

Although deeply centered around Levine's Somatic Experiencing framework, the Body-First Healing Roadmap will introduce you to a combination of modalities. Top-down approaches will include psychoeducation and attachment therapy. Bottom-up approaches will include Polyvagal Theory and nervous system regulation, Somatic Experiencing, and somatic IFS therapy.

Top-Down Approaches to Healing

When we talk about top-down versus bottom-up therapeutic approaches, most people believe that top-down simply means healing from the brain and bottom-up means healing from the body. Although not too far off, the technical differentiation is based on the region of the brain that is being targeted during the therapy.

The mainstream therapeutic approach to trauma takes a top-down stance, suggesting that treatment should start at the top of the brain in the neocortex, aka your "talking" or "thinking brain." This is where logical thought, rationale, and explicit or narrative memories are found. This is often referred to as your conscious or cortical brain. On the other hand, somatic healing predominantly focuses on the subcortical or subconscious parts of the brain, which we'll discuss more soon.

As I mentioned in the previous chapter, research shows that exposure-based or recall therapy, which guides us back into the painful memories of the past, can actually exacerbate symptoms of PTSD. Why? Because when you rehash or talk about a traumatic experience, the amygdala, which is your brain's threat or fear center, becomes activated. The amygdala turns on when your nervous system senses that it's in danger. When this happens, it turns off the prefrontal cortex—the thinking, talking, rational, remembering part of the brain *essential* for talk therapy. So it can be said that if the goal of healing is to get you unstuck from your chronic dysregulated state of survival, then continually recalling and talking about the past can do the opposite.

Many of my clients have done exposure-based or recall therapy for years in the hopes that it would effectively treat their trauma. Sadly, most of them told me that talking about their trauma left them feeling stuck, defeated, or worse. When I explain to them that starting with the trauma itself can overwhelm and further dysregulate a person's nervous system, they sigh in relief. Their trauma had unwittingly been compounded because they hadn't yet been given a safe container in which to do the work.

In fact, the thrown-in-the-deep-end approach to healing can not only heighten symptoms, but also create a relationship of codependency whereby your therapist becomes your only lifeboat. Instead, you should first be introduced to the shallow waters, where you're gently guided and supported to swim on your own. If your therapist doesn't give you tools or practices to do on your own time, then they might not be the therapist for you. You should be working with a therapist who wants to empower you to self-heal, and who consistently reminds you that although they can be a support, you have everything inside of you to return to wholeness. In fact, I remember feeling anxious to tell a previous therapist that I was ready to leave the nest and bring our sessions to an end. Her response—"My goal as a therapist is to get you to a place where you no longer need me"—reassured me that I had been in good hands.

Here are some questions I considered when I was looking for the right therapist:

Are my therapy sessions empowering me?

Am I getting workable strategies to integrate the healing on my own?

Do they rush into the trauma of the past, or do they take intentional time to build trust, rapport, and safety with me first?

Do they allow me to feel, or do they just guide me back into my thoughts?

You may be wondering if therapy is beneficial for you. My answer is that it's less of an "if" question and more of a "when" and "how" question. Many people have been incredibly successful with therapy when they start first with the body and nervous system and then move on to the cognitive and meaning-making piece of the pie.

WHY MINDFULNESS PRACTICES MIGHT NOT BE ENOUGH

"Change your thoughts, change your life." That's a saying familiar to anyone who spends time in the wellness arena—the modalities and practices centered around mindfulness, conscious awareness, and meditation. However, this well-intentioned tagline couldn't be farther from the truth. Because if your body and nervous system aren't on board, you're just going to stay stuck. The reason why meditation, mindfulness, and positive affirmations aren't enough for nervous system regulation is because you are throwing a thinking solution at a feeling problem. From a Somatic Experiencing approach, we consider that too much talking, thinking, or hanging around in our mind actually can be a management strategy to avoid feeling.

Now that's not to say that mindfulness practices don't have their place. However, when the body and subconscious mind are dismissed, these practices are simply temporary solutions. As we often say, *your state creates your story*. In other words, whatever nervous system state you're in is going to create the stories and the thoughts in your mind.

When my nervous system state was locked in that fight response after the assault, I was angry at the world. I was angry in my relationships. I was angry at work. I was angry at the TV. I was angry at the sky. I was a bitter, angry person. No matter how much positive thinking or meditation or controlled breathing or yoga or anger management classes I tried, those angry thoughts still came to the surface. Yes, I could change my thought patterns temporarily. But because all that pent-up adrenaline and cortisol and survival hormones were still trapped within my physiology, I was like a pressure cooker, with no way to let off the steam in a healthy and productive way. I was either going to implode or explode—and explode I did.

The methodology here again comes back to *when* and *how* you're using these practices. For instance, mindfulness and yoga and controlled breathing are very effective for anchoring or grounding yourself in calm and presence after you've experienced and expelled the charge of survival hormones. But because people assume that the first step in regulation is calming down, rather than expressing and releasing the stuck survival charge bellowing like mad below the surface, they often fall short in these practices. If you find that mindfulness and meditation aren't working for you, it might simply be a further invitation to get out of your mind and into your body more.

Bottom-Up Approaches to Healing

Today's research estimates that 95 percent of our brain's activity is subconscious, meaning that the vast majority of our thoughts, behaviors, and emotions are informed by the 95 percent of brain activity that exists below the neocortex.[1] As you'll see in the rest of the book, Somatic Experiencing takes a bottom-of-the-brain-up approach to trauma.

Within the Somatic Experiencing framework, we start with the subcortical (subconscious) areas of the brain—specifically the limbic system (mammalian/emotional brain) and brain stem (reptilian/survival brain) that govern our body and nervous system. Again, because trauma also shuts down the rational, higher-functioning parts of the brain and triggers physical responses, we start with those somatic imprints. The language of these subcortical structures are impulse, sensation, feeling, and emotion, so that's the language we explore. Only after finding regulation and safety through the body can we then gain effective access to the meaning-making power of the neocortex. That's why body-*first* is in the title of this book, not body-*only*.

To begin learning the language of your unique nervous system and body, start the daily commitment of "Tracking Your Nervous System," detailed on page 269 in Appendix A. I've always shared with clients that if they could do one thing that would bring the most impact to their healing, tracking would be it. And those who've worked with me or graduated from the Body-First Healing Program agree.

Debunking Misconceptions about Trauma

Can trauma be completely healed? What if I can't remember my trauma? These, and other questions are commonly asked by new clients or people curious about somatic healing. Let's explore these concepts together.

Can Trauma Be Completely Healed?

The concept of being "healed" depends on your own definition of the term. If you hold the view that healing grants you the ability to never again be *triggered* or *bothered* by past experiences, then no, you cannot be fully healed. This is because your body and nervous system will never forget the traumatic experiences of the past and will always warn you when it believes that potential threat is happening again. But—and this is an enormous *but*—the intensity of the triggers (aka activation) can minimize greatly over time. As you regulate your nervous system and expand your window of tolerance to stress, what might have once felt especially triggering can become much easier to process over time. Think of it this way: The trigger or discomfort or emotion isn't too big; your current capacity or ability to experience that discomfort is too small. So if you can instead hold the view that trauma is less about getting over something completely and more about getting better at being with it, then yes, you can fully heal. Ultimately, it's not about extinguishing the trauma, it's about *relating* to that trauma in a more resilient and regulated way.

What If I Can't Remember the Trauma?

I hear this a lot. And my response is always that *remembering* is not the same thing as *recovering*. And although we may not explicitly remember the trauma, our body implicitly remembers it.

Here's an example: Perhaps you experienced abuse as a child, but you have no narrative recollection of it; you've just been told by family members. This trauma shows up today in your reluctance to be emotionally or physically close or intimate in relationships due to increased fear of getting hurt or taken advantage of. Underneath these avoidant patterns is the fact that you were never able to fight or flee, and instead your nervous system went into a freeze or shutdown state, whereby you disconnect or isolate from others. An eventual goal in your healing could be to explore somatic practices that gently promote defensive responses through reaffirming healthy aggression and boundaries (the fight response) in the present, which was suppressed or thwarted in the past. As we'd work together, the adrenaline and cortisol that have been stuck and overwhelming your system would be released in the here and now—giving way to regulation and slowly moving you out of that shutdown or disconnected state.

Even if you don't have conscious memory of something that happened to you, you can still work with the implicit or subconscious memory and the impulses of your nervous system to allow you to do now what you couldn't do back then. The topic of memory will be deeply examined and explored in chapter 4.

Healing Imperfectly

Another valuable distinction to make is that healing will never look "perfect" in the way that our society conditions us to see it. Why? Because you will still get triggered, because your nervous system isn't rational, and because there's no such thing as a "bad nervous system state" (we'll get to that later in the book), which means that we'll still have times when we overreact, get overwhelmed, shut down, isolate, go numb, and more. First, these patterns were habitual, which means they'll take time to remove as our default. Second, sometimes circumstances call for these kind of nervous system responses.

On those hard days, when it feels messy and like it's all too much, how can you offer yourself grace? I often encourage clients to reframe such words as *regression* and *relapse* as just simply *being human*. Healing is ten steps forward, three steps back, and repeat. Again and again. The true testament of healing is holding compassion for yourself on the days you move backward, while remembering that you're still seven steps farther than you were last time.

Mainstream Medicine Is Starting to Catch Up

"Well, if Somatic Experiencing is so effective, why isn't it more mainstream? Why isn't it talked about?" I hear these questions all the time, and my very honest answer is two-fold.

First, follow the money.

Perhaps you've heard the term *sick care* used when describing the model of the health-care *industry* in America today. Sick care can be attributed to a health-care system that focuses on treating illness or symptoms while ignoring their root cause. We also can think of this as symptom management, a Band-Aid approach, or an allopathic model, which is the basis for conventional Western or modern medicine today. An ideal health-care system would be a more integrated model focused on prevention. It would consider not only the symptoms, but also the direct causes, as well as being dedicated to keeping the population healthy.

A sick-care industry, though, is much more profitable, as the main objective is to provide as many billable services as possible rather than ensure a healthy outcome for the patient. Our sick-care industry today is flourishing—Americans now spend a third of their household income on health care, and the average family of four spends $22,000 on it annually[2]—a dramatic rise from twenty years ago. It's a big business. So why would an insurance company approve a recovery approach it knows will be a short-term service that reintroduces you to the innate tools you already possess within your biology to heal on your own? Somatic Experiencing doesn't include profitable medications, interventions, or procedures, and it doesn't require a lifelong diagnosis.

That's reason number one of my two-fold response. Reason number two is pretty straightforward: it takes eighteen to twenty years for proven science to be incorporated into mainstream medical practice—practically an entire generation. (Physicians who once would have rolled their eyes at the methodology of traditional Chinese medicine now routinely refer their patients for acupuncture treatments, for example.) As renowned author and family physician Dr. Mark Hyman once shared, "Psychiatry is in the dark ages, and we have really crummy ways of dealing with trauma." We're seeing this same evolution in the trauma recovery space today. I've heard from countless seasoned and licensed therapists who are now adding somatic therapy to their practice; these same practitioners received less than ten hours of education on trauma when they were getting their degrees. And what about education surrounding nervous system regulation and body-oriented healing practices? That's still catching up, too.

The good news is that as more studies are being done, the decades-old science behind Somatic Experiencing and body-oriented healing is finally starting to emerge in the mainstream as the new frontier of trauma recovery. It's a path forged by few, but one that reaches deeper than any methodology we've long settled for. Whenever I hear a frustrated "Why are we not taught this? It would help so much!" from clients or colleagues, my simple response is that it's never too late to take a somatic approach to trauma and healing. The body always remembers.

CHAPTER 3

Defining Trauma

E arly on in my own recovery I often found ways, without even recognizing it, to downplay my own suffering. In hindsight, it was a brilliant coping strategy. Until, of course, it wasn't. By minimizing my trauma and keeping it small, it was stashed out of view and off the radar, but it was still there. I did this in a number of ways.

You could hear it, first, in the way I spoke about my past.

With my brother's death, it was: "Oh, it happened a long time ago."

With the abandonment by my biological father, it was: "Well, but my stepdad is like my real dad. So it's made no difference to me."

With my assault, it was: "But that experience gave me purpose. It catapulted me into a beautiful career path in the violence prevention and recovery space."

Regardless of whether these things were true, they negated the very real and very valid pain that I experienced.

There were other ways I minimized my trauma. Like in my relentless pursuit to put myself in the middle of other people's healing. It certainly isn't bad to want to help others, but for me, I was subconsciously doing it as a way to distract myself from my own pain. It started when I began volunteering as a counselor at a summer camp for bereaved children at the age of sixteen, shortly after my brother passed away. For years that followed, supporting others was one of my most effective coping strategies. And even more, I'd eventually also use the trauma of others as validation that mine "wasn't so bad."

Ultimately, to prove this point to myself, I was drawn to some of the darkest corners of the globe. After graduating from college with a degree in photojournalism and a minor in women's studies, with concentrations in gender-based violence and violence prevention, I set out on a global quest to "heal the world," while at the same time neglecting myself. Over the course of five years, as a domestic and international conflict and social justice documentary photographer, I bore witness to the kind of trauma my brain couldn't comprehend. Working assignments for months at a time, I became deeply embedded in the lives and experiences of the people whose heart-wrenching, yet inspiring stories I illustrated—young girls saved from forced child marriage in India, orphans who lost their entire families to disease and famine in Uganda, homeless camps in the inner cities in the United States, and more.

I remember one woman in particular, Abina, who I became especially close with while working with a Rape Crisis Center in South Africa. At the time, Abina, a four-time survivor of sexual assault who had escaped an abusive home, was living with her four children in a safe house, sheltered away from the violence and terror her husband had subjected each of them to for years.

I was always intentional about first building rapport and trust with the people whose lives I was documenting. I'd leave my camera at home for the first two weeks of any new assignment so we could simply spend time getting to know one another. When I first met Abina, we attended church together, had meals, took her children to school, and certainly cried together. Despite her experiences, Abina had a remarkably hopeful outlook on life. She exuded the purest of joy, even in the darkest of circumstances.

When I look back on those few months I spent in South Africa, I can't help but think about Abina. Yet what's also etched in my mind is the time I spent in isolation when I wasn't working. The routine stops at the liquor store on the way home from work. And the entire bottles of alcohol I'd consume to escape the deafening silence of my own pain. Alone and numb.

Here I was, acting like a real-life Mother Teresa to the outside world, but I was drinking heavily and completely disconnected from myself.

And then there was Abina, who had faced the worst that this world has to offer, but like many of the people whose stories I captured through my lens, she was seemingly okay. Maybe even more than okay. She had found a way to make space for her grief when it surfaced, to cry and express it and let it move through. And when the wave of grief would retract, it would reveal astonishing joy and aliveness. Abina could look her trauma in the face with both radical acceptance and resilience, while I, on the other hand, had ventured as far as the other side of the world to avoid my own. On paper, she and the others I met certainly "had it worse" than me, in terms of the horrors they'd gone through. Yet I seemed to be the one who was actually worse off in the end.

This was a profound revelation in my recovery. Trauma isn't about the experience or the event; it's more about how we hold it, or refuse to hold it, inside.

In this chapter, we will delve into a deeper understanding of what trauma is, so you can identify the imprints of your own trauma and begin to glimpse your road to recovery.

What Actually Is Trauma?

Trauma is any event or experience that's too overwhelming for the nervous system. This overwhelm can be described as anything that's either too much, too fast, too soon, or not enough. It's in these experiences that the nervous system isn't prepared to cope.

Imagine your nervous system as a security system, always working in the background (aka your subconscious) to protect you from anything it *perceives* is not safe. When your system becomes overwhelmed, it means that there's a lack of safety (either emotional or physical) available to disarm the security system. This results in what you could consider a faulty alarm, one that's either constantly signaling for danger when it's no longer there, or not signaling for danger when it is present.

It's important to note that what feels "safe" or "unsafe" is *relative* to each unique nervous system. In other words, what feels traumatic to one person might not feel traumatic to another. Here's an example:

Jimmy and Stevie are eight-year-old neighbors who go to the same school. Jimmy lives in a home in which both parents are consistently home, are responsive and supportive when Jimmy has big emotions, and are able to model healthy expression and regulation themselves. Stevie lives in a home in which one parent travels for work most of the time while the other struggles with addiction, explosive rage, and periods of complete withdrawal.

One day, on the school bus, Jimmy and Stevie are both bullied by the same bully. The boys are called the same names, and the bully swings the same punches at each. Jimmy and Stevie will have the same traumatic experience, right? Not so much. Here's why . . .

When Jimmy gets home after school, bruised and upset, he's met with empathy and compassion from his parents. They allow him to cry, they hold and comfort him, they validate his pain, and then they assure him they'll contact the school right away to get this resolved. He feels seen and supported. He feels *safe*. Safe enough for his nervous system to disarm and come back into a place of "deactivation" and regulation. When Jimmy is an adult, this experience might feel like just a blip in his past, and it won't be recognized as traumatic.

Stevie has a different experience. He arrives home after school, also bruised and upset. But Stevie isn't met by an empathetic witness. Stevie comes home to find one parent gone on another long work trip, and another parent who's passed out, intoxicated, on the couch. He wakes the parent and shares about his experience through tears. Stevie's big emotions provoke an irate response. "Oh, get OVER it! Take those tears to someone who cares! Stop being a baby. Stick up for yourself next time! Now go to your room." Still visibly shaken and upset, Stevie retreats to his bedroom, where his cries are muffled in exile. There's no safety to be found. No deactivation or disarming of his nervous system. Stevie remains stuck in survival. As an adult, he looks back on this experience with deep pain and recognizes it as a traumatic moment in his past.

Ultimately, if, after the initial trauma is over, your body still doesn't *feel* safe, then your nervous system will remain armored.

Not Enough

So many of us prescribe to the view that trauma must be a swift and cataclysmic event, one that leaves glaring craters in the aftermath that simply can't be overlooked. My first seasons of healing in conventional therapy focused on such events—the traumatic experiences that were visible enough to be put on a timeline. Losing my brother when I was fifteen, and the assault at twenty. These were the sufferings that were more obvious to the eye. The ones that were *too much, too fast, too soon.*

However, this rigid perspective dismisses a more nuanced pain we may experience in relationships or at moments in life when we're met with *not enough* of something. For me, this included *not enough* presence from my parents—I had a biological father who made the choice to never be a part of my life and a mother who put work above all else, even living in a separate state for her job three days a week for eleven years of my upbringing.

I also was met with *not enough* empathy following my assault—instead, there were underlying (and sometimes blatant) suggestions of blame as well as criticism and judgment from friends, family members, first responders, and my community. A few days after my assault, the police were aggressively following each lead to find and apprehend my perpetrator, but he was still on the loose. While my family and I sat in limbo, news crews began arriving at my home as my information had been accidentally leaked in a press release by an intern. Worried for my safety, my parents sent me from Indianapolis to Seattle to stay with family. Before leaving, they urged me to stay offline and avoid reading the news stories about the assault. And of course, when your parents tell you to do something, you tend to do the opposite. Or is that just me?

What I gathered from reading the police statements, articles, and comments on the stories left by those in my community was that I was responsible for what happened to me.

The last sentence in one article included a quote from the local police sergeant: "This rape holds valuable lessons. She was more afraid of feeling guilty and hurting his feelings, but instead, put herself in harm's way," he said. "She was uncomfortable about this situation from the beginning, and she really didn't want to give him a ride and probably should have trusted her instincts at that point."[1]

That was the final takeaway: I should have made different choices, and it was my fault. I was the one who had a lesson to learn, not the man who so violently took advantage of me.

Here were some of the comments that followed the piece:

She let him into her car, what did she expect?!

Didn't her mother teach her not to talk to strangers?!

I heard she was drinking that night.

Likewise, in the crucial moments after the attack, I didn't receive the support I so desperately needed. I remember the distrustful attitude of the responding officer who took my witness statement from the hospital bed. "And how much did you have to drink last night?" he asked. "Well, why did you let him into your car?" When I got home that night, I vividly recall stumbling into my front door. I was bruised and battered with an injured jaw and markings all over my face and body from the impact of my assailant's fists and the tire iron he used to beat me. I remember waking up my best friend who was asleep on my couch, and screaming at her in utter disbelief and pain. Her response was the ultimate blow, the knockout punch. All she could say to me was, "Go to bed, sleep it off, and we'll talk in the morning."

I can still feel the rage from my mother as we drove home from the hospital the next day: "We taught you better than this! Why did you let him into your car?! Why were you drinking?!"

Not enough.

What I remember most from that horrible night and the days that followed isn't the event itself, but the *aftermath*. The lack of compassionate support. The feeling of isolation and shame that festered into a self-hatred that nearly took my life years later. Not enough compassion, not enough comfort, not enough validation. Not enough safety to heal the imprint of what was done to me. It was this not-enough-ness that catapulted me into years of self-destructive behaviors—eating disorders, binge drinking, self-harm, and more.

The moments of not-enough-ness can be just as devastating as events that feel like too much, too fast, too soon. And in fact, because they're often overlooked in favor of the more glaring experiences and left untreated, they also tend to create more debilitating and extreme symptoms, including anxiety, depression, fatigue, chronic pain and illness, and addiction, to name a few.

Naming Your Trauma

People categorize or label trauma in many ways. And although it's not necessary for healing, and I never encourage anyone to put their trauma into a box, it also can be supportive to identify where your experience falls on the spectrum. (Be sure to visit the Reflection at the end of the chapter to start the process of Naming Your Trauma.)

As we've discussed, people often assume that trauma stems only from a specific catastrophic event. However, because trauma is not found in the event, but rather in the nervous system trauma also can be experienced through seemingly smaller moments that can be just as devastating. This is especially true for young children, whose nervous systems are still developing and, therefore, have a greater likelihood of being overwhelmed.

These days, some people in the mental health community refer to "big *T* trauma" and "little *t* trauma," the idea being that some types of experiences are more detrimental than others. Yet what we must remember is that what might feel like a catastrophic big *T* trauma to one nervous system, might feel like a small little *t* trauma to another. Labeling our trauma in this way can feel invalidating.

Instead of labeling what's big and not big, we can understand the spectrum of trauma better by looking at more objective factors. These factors include whether we experienced the trauma directly or indirectly, as well as the length and frequency of the trauma.

Direct Trauma

Direct trauma is experienced directly through us. In the next section, we'll explore the more nuanced experiences of indirect trauma. For now, let's look at the three types of direct trauma.

Acute Trauma

Acute trauma is what we most commonly envision when referring to trauma. It's the shock trauma that happens out of nowhere. It's the in-your-face kind of trauma that's sensationalized in books and on our TV screens. Acute trauma happens due to a single and short-lasting *event* that has a clear beginning, middle, and end. Some examples of acute trauma include (but of course aren't limited to): a motor vehicle accident, a sexual assault, a breakup, a betrayal, a death or illness of a loved one, a sudden loss of a job, a natural disaster, a life-threatening diagnosis, a medical trauma, an attack, and more.

Chronic

Chronic trauma is the not-so-obvious trauma that lurks in the corners of our subconscious. These are the experiences that are often overlooked, typically because they don't fit the cultural narrative of a catastrophic event. What results is an invisible wound that eventually festers into a cascade of traumatic symptoms. Chronic trauma is defined as a single and long-lasting *experience* that happens over time. It's a season or cycle of an ongoing experience that doesn't have a particular beginning, middle, and end. It might be emotional neglect, abandonment, separation from parents, divorce, extreme poverty, living in a home with someone who has substance abuse issues, emotional or physical abuse, unhealthy relationships, bullying, war, oppression, domestic violence, mental illness in the home, and more.

Complex

Complex trauma is the newest of the three categories of direct trauma. Complex trauma refers to the exposure to multiple traumatic events or experiences that occur during an extended period and is often a combination of acute and/or chronic trauma. Although it's more commonly associated with childhood or "developmental" trauma, it also can be experienced by adults. What's most identifiable within the complex trauma experience is that there's typically a cascade of symptoms that create further trauma after the dust settles.

For example, when Shannon's spouse cheated on her, the betrayal was the root trauma, the acute trauma. Their subsequent divorce, losing her home, and a contentious custody battle over her children was also traumatic. Distraught, angry, and full of grief, Shannon didn't have the supportive coping mechanisms to deal with the overwhelm, so she resorted to heavy drinking. She eventually received a DUI and lost her job as well as custody of her children. Because her original trauma was never faced or healed, the compounding domino effect led to complex trauma.

Invalidation is often part of complex trauma. In the aftermath of the original trauma, someone may experience a lack of empathy from others—it could be someone dismissing you, not listening to you, telling you to "get over it" (like my coaches did), or not believing you. Or you may not have anyone to support you at all. This can be made worse when a medical professional, a therapist, a teacher, or a family member (supposedly there to help you), is dismissive.

In my experience, my assault was the acute trauma I had to work through. But the way others responded in the aftermath created a completely different trauma to heal. The Body-First Healing Roadmap will support you in separating and healing both the experiences of the original trauma (aka your core wound) and its aftermath.

Indirect Trauma

Perhaps you've stumbled upon this book with no explicit traumatic memories in tow. "I have all the signs and symptoms of experiencing trauma, yet I don't recall any" is a statement I hear often in my practice. Although it frequently boils down to my clients realizing they did in fact experience trauma after learning the true meaning of trauma and how nuanced and "non-catastrophic" it can be, there's also another simple explanation many clients come to know as well: you can experience trauma indirectly, through circumstances that happen *around* you, but not directly *to* you.

Intergenerational Trauma

The apple doesn't fall far from the tree, especially when trauma is involved. The trauma of our ancestors is our scar to bear as well. A vast collection of research has uncovered that we inherit legacies of survival from earlier generations, encoded in everything from gene expression and hormones to everyday language, impulse, and behavior, all of which contribute to our overall mental, emotional, and physical health.

Slavery, war, genocide, colonization, immigration, family secrets or shame, an epidemic, the Depression—the impact of historical moments like these can be passed down in our belief systems or actually *transmitted* through DNA for up to three, or perhaps even more, generations.

Also commonly referred to as "epigenetics," studies show us that our genetics and our unique nervous systems are particularly shaped by the experience of family who came before us. In other words, alterations in our epigenetics can be passed down from one generation to another, effectively giving parents a way to prime their children for a particular environment or threat—known as "transgenerational genetic inheritance."

In an epigenetics study conducted in 2013, Emory University researchers Brian Dias and Kerry Ressler exposed a group of mice to a particular smell of cherry blossoms while simultaneously giving them a mild shock to the foot, creating a conditioned startle or fear response when the mice would smell this odor. However, this learned fear didn't end with this group of mice. The researchers were astonished to find that not only did the immediate offspring (children) of these mice also fear the smell of cherry blossoms, even though they were *never shocked themselves*, but also their offspring (grandchildren) had a startled fear response when the smell was presented. What's more, they found that these descendants also had inherited structural changes to their olfactory systems; they had enhanced neuron receptors in their nose to detect that exact odor—better priming them for survival.[2]

There have been countless human studies on intergenerational trauma in the past few decades as well, like the well-known Holocaust studies done by Rachel Yehuda and her research team at New York's Mount Sinai Hospital. The research revealed that descendants of Holocaust survivors had altered and elevated levels of stress hormones compared to those who were not the descendants of Holocaust survivors.[3]

Although generational trauma shows the profound and lasting imprint of trauma, it also reveals the positive impact we can make on future generations when we heal in the present.

Vicarious or Secondary Trauma

Another category of indirect trauma is vicarious or secondary trauma. This occurs when we care for, hear about, or witness the trauma of others in a way that feels too overwhelming for our own nervous system, causing us to take on the similar symptoms of those who experienced the trauma directly.

This can happen in many ways. It could be when we're exposed to disturbing images or videos on social media or in the news. Or when we drive by a horrific accident shortly after it happened and unwittingly see the aftermath. Or when we witness abuse in the home, even though it's not directed at us. It also could happen when we are exposed to the trauma of others on a consistent basis because of our profession. This is common with first responders, therapists, social workers, military members, and more.

Vicarious or secondary trauma is also where collective trauma resides—when a traumatic event affects a large group of people, including entire societies or communities. Some examples include terrorist attacks, pandemics and epidemics, recessions, genocide, religious persecution, racial trauma, misogyny, natural disasters, and more. The concept of vicarious or secondary trauma highlights the interconnectedness of our traumas—and how these experiences don't have to isolate us, but perhaps can connect us and bring us together.

DEVELOPMENTAL TRAUMA

Developmental trauma, which we'll explore later in this book, is another term used for childhood trauma, which occurs through sensitive periods of infant and child development. The name is attributed to the ways in which trauma directly disrupts and influences development in relation to sensory development, attachment development, emotional and behavioral regulation, cognition, and development of identity or self. Children's young brains and nervous systems don't yet have the mature tools and cognition adults have to adapt to stress, which leaves young children particularly vulnerable to the effects of trauma and its more long-standing consequences. Ultimately, trauma in childhood can disrupt a person's ability to process information, which then impacts their behavior and emotional well-being.

Further evidence from the Adverse Childhood Experiences (ACE) Study also concludes that developmental trauma is often the precursor for health conditions in adulthood, such as chronic illness, disease, personality and learning disorders, and more.[4] For example, one population study showed that children (under the age of eighteen) with a history of abuse or neglect have four times the increased risk of developing a personality disorder.[5] With these findings in mind, we can easily say that childhood trauma should be considered when treating developmental symptoms or disorders.

Reflection: Naming Your Trauma

As you begin to take a personal inventory of the possible traumatic experiences in your life, there may be some that are more visible and others that perhaps you're just now considering were too much, too fast, too soon, or not enough for your nervous system to cope with. We'll be exploring and identifying the exact core wounds that are still affecting you in a later chapter, but let's begin to get curious about what you may discover:

1. Which of these categories do you feel you fall into more? Or can you relate to multiple?
   » **Acute trauma:** A single, short-lasting event
   » **Chronic trauma:** A single, long-lasting experience
   » **Complex trauma:** Multiple traumas, either acute or chronic, that create a domino effect of more trauma

2. Which of these categories do you feel you fall into more? Or can you relate to both?
   » Experiences that felt like too much, too soon, or too fast. Examples include assault, abuse, bullying, war, violence, car accident, sudden loss, natural disaster, breakup, job loss, etc.
   » Experiences that felt like having not enough of something. Examples include abandonment, neglect, extreme poverty, separation from parent, divorce in childhood, oppression, etc.

3. Which of these categories do you feel you fall into more? Or can you relate to both?
   » **Direct trauma:** Experiencing trauma directly
   » **Indirect trauma:** Experiencing trauma through someone else, including intergenerational trauma, vicarious or secondary trauma, or collective trauma.

CHAPTER 4

Traumatic Memory

Trauma comes back as a reaction, not a memory.
—Bessel van der Kolk

I n his groundbreaking book, *The Body Keeps the Score*, Bessel van der Kolk poignantly shares, "The nature of trauma is that you have no recollection of it as a *story*. The nature of traumatic experience is that the brain doesn't allow a story to be created." He adds, "Trauma comes back as a *reaction*, not a memory."

As you'll come to deeply understand in this chapter, trauma leaves all of us with indelible imprints that can continue to haunt us, regardless of whether or not we can consciously recall it all. Although the memory centers of your brain may not have been present to witness the suffering (we'll dive into that science soon), the body was always there to feel, sense, impulsively react, and experience it all. In other words, you might not remember what happened, but your body still remembers how it *felt*. And when reminded of, or triggered by, these somatic imprints or "felt memories," your body instinctually refers to the ancient wisdom of your nervous system's reaction at that time—fight, flight, shutdown, freeze, or fawn.

Preverbal Traumatic Memory

The room began to fade to black and back to light as I tried my best to fix my tear-filled eyes on the leaves of the southern magnolia tree swaying outside the window. I was curled up in the fetal position on a massage table, wrapped up in a cocoon of weighted blankets and pillows. My somatic therapist sat beside me, out of view, but I could sense her there. My breath felt shallow, my brain foggy, and my limbs internally cold yet externally numb.

"What might you notice now?" she softly asked.

I paused, taking a moment to find my words. "I feel dizzy, like I'm floating away."

Another pause, "Yes, that makes sense," she replied gently. "This could be the drugs or toxins that you experienced in the womb, the methamphetamine, that's causing the loopy and leaving feeling. Or," she added slowly, "because your little body couldn't mount a defense during this distressing experience, a state of shutdown and dissociation was your only coping mechanism."

The shallow tears that pooled in the corners of my eyes flooded over as an unexpected surge of grief, loneliness, and sadness emerged. I shuddered and hugged my knees tighter into my chest. The tears spilled out as I sobbed and brought my hand to my heart, which was literally aching. I rode that wave of activation until my breath started to catch back up to me, my muscles began to soften, and my vision could reorient to the environment around me.

"You see, your body knows exactly what to do," my therapist said encouragingly. "And as you begin to slowly come back into the present moment, and back into your body, I'm curious—would it be supportive for you if I applied just a little pressure with my hands to the tops of your feet? To really help you to feel grounded?"

I quickly (and surprisingly) responded, "That would be wonderful, thank you." We sat there for a time, saying nothing, just feeling deeper into the safety of the moment we were in. As our session came to a close, I noticed a remarkable contrast from how I felt when I'd first walked into that room. I now felt lighter, more peaceful, hopeful, and empowered by my seemingly innate ability to be with intense moments of pain and to work through them.

I was in my late twenties at the time, and this was my first somatic session exploring the trauma I had experienced while in the womb. I had originally begun working with my therapist to address the ongoing sense of unworthiness and fear of abandonment that seemed to rule my life. These feelings had impacted my ability to articulate my inner world, to assert my wants and needs, and to show up comfortably in my own skin—and had resulted in crippling imposter syndrome, unhealthy codependency, severe social anxiety that I could only mask by consuming copious alcoholic beverages to "loosen" up, as well as an extreme eating disorder, among other things. Unable to pinpoint the source of this feeling of incompleteness within, and no longer willing to remain estranged from myself and the world around me, I leaned into my somatic therapist for support.

I was shocked when our work together eventually traced back to my birth trauma, a type of developmental trauma often overlooked in diagnoses of mental health conditions such as depression or anxiety. I had always assumed that surely it was my father's absence, or the death of my brother, that left me so "broken and wounded." Yet it was the trauma in utero and my subsequent entry into the world, when I was forcibly removed from my mother at birth (and was kept separated from her while in foster care for the first few crucial months of my life), that marred me with visible distress for years to come.

I've since gathered that I was the "easy baby" in comparison to my siblings, who required more attention and support. Yet in hindsight, I believe that in my case, *easy* could be translated as *detached*. Because, you see, babies aren't supposed to be easy. It's developmentally appropriate for them to show big emotions, to express their wants and desires, to cry for their caregivers, to whine when they're upset, and to test boundaries to assert their concept of self.

Developmental Trauma

The early months of a child's life are critical for developing a healthy attachment foundation, or a feeling of security that follows a child through life. (I'll discuss this more fully in the next chapter.) But when infants are separated from their birth mothers, like I was, they feel threatened, which in turn imprints feelings of unsafety in their minds and bodies. These implicit/body memories linger, shaping their adaptive reactions to the world around them and manifesting as anguishing mental and physical symptoms carried into adulthood—anxiety, obsessive-compulsive disorder (OCD), depression, addiction, and chronic pain being a few examples. One defining aspect of these early experiences is that they are preverbal, so we can't articulate them as narratives. For this reason, we may not recognize them as sources of trauma or link our suffering to these formative moments.

Sadly, these are the unhealed wounds that many of us unknowingly walk around with today. Developmental trauma casts a long shadow over a person's life, and it exists beyond conscious memory. The stress hormones unleashed during these early experiences shape the trajectory of our future development, influencing our nervous system and how we navigate the world. Such trauma could potentiate the perfect environment for a host of challenges, from learning disabilities, to allergies, and beyond.

For those haunted by developmental trauma, which occurs from the period of conception until a child develops verbal skills around the age of two or three, the journey toward healing begins with forging a sanctuary of safety within oneself. In conventional talk therapy, therapists guide patients through the labyrinth of their past, uncovering the roots of their present-day symptoms and struggles. But how do you address wounds predating language and verbal memory itself? Somatic Experiencing Practitioners, like myself, embark on this journey alongside our clients with the aim to create a sense of safety and ease within the nervous system in the *present*.

In the weeks and months that followed my somatic therapy session, I observed that same ease I had felt at the end of the session. There was a noticeable difference in my ability to manage emotions, communicate my boundaries, and remain more present and embodied in my day-to-day life. I felt secure, empowered, and, more importantly, *safe* with myself and within my body, for perhaps the first time.

Post-Traumatic Stress Reactions

As *The Body Keeps the Score* and other well-regarded books on trauma, such as *The Body Remembers: The Psychophysiology of Trauma and Trauma Treatment* by Babette Rothschild, illuminate, trauma is remembered, stored, and relived through body memory, or implicit memory. Although these books introduced the mainstream to an entirely new concept—that trauma resides in our somatic experience, wedged deep within the body—these findings have been studied and researched for more than a century. In 1889, pioneering French psychologist, physician, philosopher, and psychotherapist Pierre Janet, published *L'Automatisme Psychologique*, which systematically studied the psychological process of dissociation.[1] His findings highlighted the crucial differences between ordinary and traumatic memory, proposing that traumatic memories are split off (dissociated) from consciousness and instead stored as sensory perceptions, affect/emotional states, and behavioral reenactments in our subconscious (or unconscious) mind. And as world-renowned researcher and author Dr. Joe Dispenza puts it, "Your *body* is your subconscious mind."

These behavioral reenactments or "reactions," as van der Kolk suggests, can present themselves in subtle or more severe ways. They can show up in our everyday behaviors. Like perhaps how we avoid eye contact because, as a baby, the eyes of our caregivers were filled with rage, anxiety, or detachment—a threatening sensory experience that taught us as an infant that it's safer to look away.

These reactions also can show up in the way we respond to stress or how we manage what triggers or activates us. Perhaps you've heard stories of survivors of abuse, violence, war, or motor vehicle accidents who have no conscious recollection of the experience at all, yet still become suddenly overcome with debilitating emotions, sensations, and physical reactions when a sensory experience triggers them. For example, in his book *The Traumatic Neuroses of War*, Abram Kardiner described how numerous veteran patients who could recall little to no memory of their war experience (war amnesia, they used to call it) would have panic attacks and flashbacks of being back in the battle trenches when they'd take the subway in New York City and enter the tunnels.

Or maybe you recognize this experience in yourself. This could happen when someone raises their voice at a sports game and you immediately feel anxiety and constriction in your muscles as you hold your breath, all because your body is subconsciously remembering the familiar tone of your father's violent screams hurled at your mother, while you (a toddler) and your siblings hid in a closet—memories that you were too young and traumatized to remember, but that your body still *reacts* to. In this moment, you might not recognize that you're being triggered by an unconscious memory. Therefore, the feelings and physical reactions that this memory engenders may seem confusing, irrational, or incongruous to the present situation. I see this often in my practice with clients, and I even notice it within my own experience today, when reactions occur yet there seems to be no conscious reason to suspect they're linked to past experiences.

For example, years ago I had a Somatic Experiencing client who had a debilitating fear of driving on the highway and opted to stay only on main roads and side streets whenever she drove. This was a management strategy she used to avoid the feeling of unsafety. This made getting around difficult, of course, and the fact that the client had no rational understanding of where this anxiety came from made it all that much more challenging for her. Not only did she feel "crazy," but she also expressed her husband's growing frustration with her worsening fear after they had children. It was putting a strain on her well-being, on her marriage, and on her kids.

Although it's not always necessary to pinpoint the original trauma, or core wound, during somatic sessions, when we were working together, we eventually stumbled upon the fact that her fear was actually of semitrucks. When she was just a few months old, she and her mother experienced an accident on the highway when a semi slid on ice and swiped their car off the road. Although she couldn't recall the experience, her body remembered, and it made sure to instinctively remind her of the potential danger. Our work of uncoupling the fearful association between semitrucks and danger, as well as cultivating tools to help her *feel* safe within a car, made all the difference. It didn't take long for her to be able to sit in the passenger seat while her husband drove on the highway. After that, they were able to do the same with the kids in the car as well. And in less than six months, she was behind the wheel and driving on the highway herself with ease.

Ultimately, if trauma comes back as a reaction, then we could easily say that our reactions are always telling us a story. So instead of giving way to self-judgment or criticism of these implicit reactions and impulses, hurling the *What's wrong with me?* question at ourselves, could we instead get curious with *What happened to me?* This compassionate reframe can support us in managing the reactions that show up in our daily lives, like anxiety, depression, OCD, avoidance, isolation, and more.

What if what we often and quickly chalk up to diagnosis or disorder is merely the brain's and the body's brilliant way of *reacting* to stress, post-trauma? So instead of obsessive-compulsive *disorder*, could we consider this as an adaptive obsessive-compulsive *reaction*? Instead of generalized anxiety *disorder*, could we consider this as an adaptive generalized anxiety *reaction*? And instead of post-traumatic stress *disorder*, could we consider this as a post-traumatic stress *reaction*?

Explicit Versus Implicit Memory

To truly understand the remembrance of trauma, we must first understand the basics of memory—more specifically, explicit conscious memory and implicit unconscious memory.

Explicit Memory

Explicit memory is often described as verbal or declarative memory of information that can be consciously recalled. More simply, *explicit* memory can be *explained*. What we commonly consider memory is explicit memory, like "I went fishing with my grandpa when I was nine years old. It was a beautiful summer day. He was wearing his favorite bucket cap for good luck, and I caught my first bass!"

There are two subtypes of explicit memory:

- **Semantic memory:** The memory of general knowledge, facts, and concepts
- **Episodic memory:** The memory of personal experiences and events

Explicit memory is predominantly stored in the brain structure known as the hippocampus and begins to develop between the ages of two and three, when the hippocampus forms. This is why we don't explicitly remember life in utero, birth, or infancy. Explicit memory provides us with the who, what, where, and when of an experience. And the *when* is an important distinction, because only explicit memories receive a time stamp or chronological encoding. This is what allows us to differentiate experiences from the past and present.

Implicit Memory

On the other hand, implicit memory, commonly considered body memory, is not consciously remembered. This is non-declarative or nonverbal memory that is stored in numerous regions of the brain, including the cerebellum, the striatum, and the amygdala. Implicit memory begins developing at seven weeks gestation. For instance, we learn the muscle memory of sucking our thumb in the womb as a way to soothe and comfort ourselves. I had a sweet sonogram of my son, Noah, sucking his thumb at the age of twenty weeks.

Just as with explicit memory, there are subtypes of implicit memory:

- **Procedural memory:** The memory of how to perform common tasks without actively thinking about it, such as muscle memory and impulse memory
- **Emotional memory:** The memory of the emotions felt during a previous experience
- **Sensory memory:** Anything related to your five senses: sight, hearing, touch, smell, and taste

Implicit memory becomes the dominant memory in these four scenarios:

1. Before the hippocampus and explicit memory develop between the ages of two and three, therefore making all preverbal memory implicit memory

2. During traumatic experiences when the survival hormone cortisol overwhelms the brain, shrinking and shutting off the hippocampus, therefore impairing explicit memory

3. When a traumatic brain injury occurs that damages the hippocampus

4. When dissociation from the mind occurs and explicit memory isn't gathered

It's important to note that unlike explicit memory, implicit memory does *not* have a time stamping or chronological encoding process that allows us to differentiate the past and present. For instance, riding a bike or brushing your teeth are tasks that carry with them no concept of time. Further, when we have an emotional memory—for example, the grief that resurfaces when remembering a loved one—that grief also has no concept of time. That's why the grief can flood us and feel just as overwhelming today as it did when that loved one passed.

As colleague and author Dr. Russell Kennedy, known as "The Anxiety MD," once shared with me, "a trigger is really just an emotional age regression."

Read that again: a trigger is really just an *emotional age regression.* When we think about this concept, as well as van der Kolk's declaration that "trauma comes back as a reaction, not as a memory," we can consider that when an implicit memory of trauma is triggered, because there is no concept of time within that emotion (whether it be shame, fear, anxiety, anger, etc.), our body and brain revert to the *emotional reaction* at the time of the original trauma. All of a sudden, our adult selves are catapulted back to the somatic and emotional experiences of the past.

HOW ARE MEMORIES FORMED?

The intricate process of memory formation begins with *encoding,* when sensory input is first processed in primary sensory areas like visual and auditory centers. This raw data is then converted or translated into cohesive memory.

Next is *storing,* when the information gets retained in memory.

Retrieval comes last, orchestrated by the prefrontal cortex and storage areas, where we can consciously re-access the memories that have been successfully encoded and stored.

Another simple way to summarize this process is converting, retaining, and recalling information.

Visible Wounds

Implicit memory also can present itself visibly in the body through our fascia, muscles, and viscera, impacting our posture, our impulses, and how our body takes up space in the world.

I remember watching a video during my Somatic Experiencing Practitioner training of Peter Levine working with a young Iraq War veteran named Ray who was injured during an improvised explosive device (IED) explosion. After waking from a coma two weeks after the incident, Ray was diagnosed with a traumatic brain injury, PTSD, chronic pain, and sudden Tourette's syndrome due to the incessant twitching his body now experienced. Levine noted in a separate interview that he was curious about Ray's Tourette's diagnosis, because this isn't often something that appears suddenly.

In the video, Levine worked with Ray's twitching response in the neck, which he ultimately concluded were the *stuck or incomplete orienting and defensive impulses* that Ray experienced as his body was lifted into the air during the blast. In other words, at the initial moment of the explosion, Ray's instinctual "startle" response was to turn his eyes, head, and neck toward the source of the threat or sound of the explosion while also pulling his shoulders up to protect himself—like a turtle going into a shell. However, within mere milliseconds, he was suddenly propelled up into the air—overwhelming his body and nervous system and causing the incomplete defensive orienting response in his neck to repeat again and again upon waking. His trauma came back as a *reaction*.

I watched while Peter eased the pace of the session and assisted Ray in finishing his disrupted orienting response to the explosion, a process meant to calm the convulsions in his head and neck. Amazingly, yet not surprisingly, it took only six Somatic Experiencing sessions for Ray's tremors and Tourette's to completely disappear. Ray shared in a later interview, "I learned to use what he taught me [the somatic tools], and use it by myself." Today, Ray often volunteers alongside Levine in the Somatic Experiencing recovery work he provides to veterans.

Ray's story reminded me of a short World War I medical film called

War Neuroses I watched as a photojournalism student while in college. The 1917 film, created by Major Arthur Hurst, documented the medical treatment provided to shell shock and war amnesia patients who'd been admitted to Seale Hayne Military Hospital in Devon, England.[2] These traumatized soldiers in particular suffered from intractable movement disorders following the war, with symptoms including staggering, shuffling, twitching, dancing, and shaking—neurological presentations that were very commonly found in these veterans.

The 2009 book *Hysterical Men: War, Psychiatry, and the Politics of Trauma in Germany, 1890–1930* by Paul Lerner described the film as such: "The bizarre, involuntary contortions of the war neurotic's body bespoke, it seemed, the hidden dangers of modern, mechanized warfare. . . . Indeed, the persistent shaking, perhaps the paradigmatic war neurosis symptom, seemed to be the inscription of the resounding, repetitious blasts on the fragile body—patients' nervous twitching mirrored the rhythm of the ceaseless, distant drum of enemy fire."

Another study of the film, this one in 2013 and conducted by researchers at the Center for Movement Disorders and Neurorestoration at the University of Florida, summarized a modern diagnosis of the soldiers' post-war injuries as "combat stress reactions" and provided these symptoms:

- Gait (walking) disorders that included imbalance, shuffling, frequent falls, staggering, and paralysis
- Abnormal postures, known as pure dystonia
- Facial spasms
- Head tremors
- Tics and convulsions
- Crippling panic attacks and anxiety
- Word blindness and deafness

After hearing Ray's story and learning the subsequent research, I couldn't help but begin to get curious about the way trauma impacted my own physical body. The noticeable shrugged and collapsed posture I had carried for years, the way I dragged and shuffled my feet when I walked, and how I rocked from side to side when I was anxious—these were all visible scars of shame. These postures and movements told the story of a young girl who felt abandoned, insecure, and disconnected, and who, as a baby, learned to self-soothe by rocking herself in the absence of her caregiver.

The more recent trauma of my assault was evident to the eye as well. Even though I was right-handed, my right side had been weaker than my left since the assault. My right shoulder even sat about two inches lower than my left. After visiting umpteen chiropractors with no relief, it wasn't until I started doing somatic work that I realized my posture was the result of an incomplete fight response during my assault. I'd been attacked on my right side, and when I tried to fight back, I was overpowered and went into a freeze response. Working with my somatic therapist to complete that defensive response on the right side of the body helped remarkably. Ultimately, your posture shows not just your history, but also what your body felt and perhaps never got to express.

A Trauma-Informed Approach to Working with Survivors

"This knowledge probably would have saved my victims from further trauma, had I known it all these years," said the detective. Sadly, I'd heard this numerous times before, from countless other victims' advocates.

I had just finished presenting a program on trauma-informed practices and memory reconsolidating for a Violent Crimes Conference in Virginia when a tenured sex crimes detective approached me to talk offstage.

It was April 2019, and by that point, I had been leading trauma-informed and forensic neurobiology trainings for law enforcement and the military for years. April had been, and always will be, a bittersweet month for me. Not only is it Sexual Assault Awareness Month, but it's also the month that my own assault happened—April 1, 2009. And every April since 2011, I've dedicated myself to speaking to audiences far and wide, as I share my story, my knowledge, and my guidance to ensure that no one else falls victim to re-traumatization in the aftermath of an assault.

I had turned on some light music on my laptop, filling the ballroom with ambient melodies as the audience of first responders, nurses, police officers, and detectives started to migrate out of the conference hall. Slowly, roughly twenty professionals fell back from the departing crowd and started to form a line behind the first detective who approached me.

"How would you all feel if we had an open discussion or Q&A together? Would that be helpful?" I asked the growing crowd. They nodded yes and made their way to the front row as I took a seat on the edge of the stage, dangling my legs over the side. Over the course of the next hour, I listened more than I talked as the group shared their reflections about the main points of my training, which are what I share with these audiences each year:

- Investigators are trained to gather testimony through narrative details: who, what, where, and when. However, traumatic memories are not stored as episodic or explicit memory. What should be explored instead are implicit memories. Questions asked could include, "Is there anything that you can sense about that experience? Is there anything that you can smell? Can you recall any colors?" Asking for sensory responses will help dislodge memory fragments that the investigators can then piece together in a nonlinear way.

- The stages of memory include encoding, storing, and then retrieving. When a victim's nervous system is regulated enough, sometimes a "memory reconsolidation" process occurs during which the narrative traumatic memory that was once not able to be retrieved comes back to the victim's conscious recollection. This can happen through fragmented memory, flashbacks, flooding, or flashbulb memories.

- Implicit memory is not stored with a time stamp. However, investigators understandably want a sequential timeline from beginning to end to make their case. Instead, when working with victims, detectives should share that it's okay if things aren't in order. Victims should never be made to feel that their story doesn't make sense, that they need to remember, or that they're being judged. This disconnects them further from both implicit and explicit memories that could be retrieved.

- How and where victims are questioned is crucial. A victim needs to be questioned in a space that feels like a safe haven, not in a cold, closed-off interrogation room. A warm, welcoming environment is essential, and so is a warm, supportive detective. A victim's frozen nervous system can only thaw out when they feel safety, trust, and empathy.

- A victim's peri-personal sphere, or the boundary map our body is always sensing, can offer further information when memories are limited.

Here's an example for context: My husband, David, was sitting in the passenger seat of a car when another car coming through an intersection hit them directly on the side where he was sitting. He was knocked unconscious during the event, but the driver was able to give witness testimony of the accident. Had David been by himself, with no recollection of what happened, an investigator questioning him could have asked, "As you imagine what the accident might have been like, do you notice any tension in your body?" To which my husband would likely respond that his muscles were bracing for impact on the right side.

When working with victims of violent crimes, it's important to gather cohesive, reputable evidence and testimony from the victim. But if law enforcement or other professionals don't enter into that process in a trauma-informed way, the victim will just shut down further.

Remembering Is Not the Same as Recovering

I've learned and seen enough professionally to conclude that when someone tells me they have a "horrible memory," I believe that what they truly mean, without recognizing it, is that they've had what their nervous system perceived to be "horrible trauma." Ironically enough, I, too, am a member of the vast club of people who don't remember much of their childhood. At the time, our brains were prioritizing surviving over remembering.

Tiny brains, little bodies, and young nervous systems that aren't yet developed or equipped to manage stress are much more vulnerable to adversity. And because children become even more vulnerable when they fight or flee, we often find that the predictable path of survival most often leads to shutdown or dissociation. In these moments, a young child will disconnect from the present, as well as disconnect from themselves, others, the world around them, and ultimately their memories. So if we were brought up in these stress-induced environments, where we lacked caretakers who were regulated themselves and where we experienced abuse, neglect, or myriad other traumatic childhood experiences (as you'll see in subsequent chapters), then not only will we have little to no narrative memory of the trauma, but we often won't remember the good things that happened either.

Many of my clients worry about the fact that they don't have conscious memories of their childhood and think this is an area they need to work on to heal. My response is to always encourage and remind them that *remembering is not the same thing as recovering.* As we've learned, trauma is not found in the event or the conscious story; it's found in the body and the instinctual reactions of the nervous system in the present day.

As Peter Levine explains, trauma lives in the survival energy and management strategies locked within our bodies in response to perceived threats or stress. We see these unconscious reactions in the ways in which we meet challenges in adulthood—the way we minimize; the way we shut down; the way we isolate, disconnect, lash out, run away, or make ourselves small. For baby Brittany, whose little body couldn't mount a defense during my own distressing prenatal experiences, a state of shutdown and disconnection became a management strategy, freezing me in a perpetual state of survival mode. This could be observed in my collapsed and slouched posture as an adult.

The essence of healing lies in expanding our capacity to be with the feelings that once felt too overwhelming, followed by discharging or releasing the trapped energy of adrenaline and cortisol in the here and now, allowing the body and the nervous system to restore equilibrium and a felt sense of safety. Somatic Experiencing facilitates this processing of experiencing, expressing, and expelling what's keeping you stuck. As you'll experience in the Body-First Healing Roadmap in part II, mastery over your body and physiology paves the way for navigating the world with newfound security. And so the good news is that even though we might not remember what happened, we can still heal and complete the stories of the past by working with the survival impulses and reactions that are showing up in the present.

Reflection: Naming Your Reactions

I invite you to reflect on the *reactions* today that tell the stories of your traumas. Without moving into the past and focusing instead on the present, what are some of the common emotional patterns, behavioral patterns, or physical observations that show up in your day-to-day life?

As an example, these are my own post-traumatic stress reactions, mentioned in this chapter:

1. **Emotions:** Shame, insecurity, fear of abandonment, and anxiety

2. **Behaviors:** Inability to articulate my inner world or assert my wants and needs, crippling imposter syndrome, unhealthy co-dependency, severe social anxiety that could be masked only by copious alcoholic beverages to "loosen" up, and disordered eating

3. **Physical observations:** Dissociation and disconnection from self, slumped posture, sluggish gait (walking style), and weakness in the right side of my body

Your Post-Traumatic Stress Reactions

1. **Emotions:**

_____

_____

2. **Behaviors:**

_____

_____

3. **Physical observations:**

_____

_____

CHAPTER 5

The Nervous System 101: Why You Make Sense

I t isn't every day that a family hiking trip on a crisp and sunny Montana day turns into a perfect example of how your nervous system protects you—and how, when faced with sudden danger, its response and how it deals with the aftermath can mean the difference between an amazing memory and years of suffering.

But that's what happened when my husband, David, and I took then-two-year-old Noah to Glacier National Park. It was the last week in May—the perfect time to visit, when the wildlife comes out of hibernation, before the summer crowds arrive, and when the waterfalls and lakes are most alive and pristine from the fresh runoff of melting snow.

Although we were avid hikers, we had originally come to the east side of the park to complete a short "beginner" hike around Swiftcurrent Lake in the Many Glacier region—a three-mile loop with little to no elevation gain that would guide us around the shores of a picturesque alpine lake with soaring mountain peaks above. It was the perfect trail for carrying a toddler on our backs for the first time. As soon as we arrived, however, we saw a crowd of spectators at the trailhead, mesmerized by one of the many hundreds of grizzly bears in the park. The bear was busy roaming the shore not far from the trailhead, and a park ranger told us that this particular grizzly had been stalking a mama moose and her twin calves who had been born a few days before. Capitalizing on the moose's exhaustion from birth, the bear had managed to grab one calf that morning and was hanging around, hoping to capture the other. My own mama heart hurt for the moose, but I also understood and accepted it was the nature of life. (Interestingly enough, the next day that mama moose successfully chased off the grizzly. A video of the confrontation went viral and was even picked up by global news networks!)

The park ranger suggested we take another trail toward Lake Josephine, which had a breathtakingly lovely roaring waterfall, but she did stress that late snowpack on the mountains was causing the bears to roam at lower elevations and reminded us to be vigilant and prepared for a potential encounter. With our bear spray holstered to our belts, we happily set out.

While we hiked through dense coniferous forest for the next hour, every now and then we'd shout, "Hey bear!" through the trees, often hearing a faint echo of "Hey bear" or the jingle of bear bells from other hikers nearby. It brought comfort to know we weren't alone, and that the other hikers were equally vigilant. By this point my back and shoulders had started to ache from the constant muscle bracing and scanning for signs of bears—not to mention that I was adamant about carrying Noah on my back in the hiking carrier because I wanted him near. It was one thing for my husband and I to hike on our own—we were used to being in proximity to wildlife—but having a toddler with us amplified our levels of adrenaline and cortisol and the overall tension of the situation.

As we stepped out from the tree line onto an open and slanted alpine meadow, I followed David's tracks in the snow, foot-by-foot. We hadn't even considered that we'd encounter snow, yet the beeline of passing hikers trekking through the mild winter terrain gave us unspoken confidence that it wasn't a big deal or unsafe in any way. By this point, David was roughly twenty steps ahead of us, and I put extra weight onto my hiking poles to keep my balance. As I ventured farther out onto the now bare yet snow-filled mountainous slope, I felt a sudden surge of wind barrel down from above, sweeping from the peak that sat over my right shoulder down to my left, where the mountain met Lake Josephine.

I heard a crack below and looked down to the shore, where I watched a chunk of snow break away from the mountain and fall into the dark water. I froze in sheer horror. I hadn't yet noticed that Lake Josephine's beautiful crystal blue water, which had captivated us on the opposite shore a scant twenty minutes before, had turned from turquoise to black.

In that moment, I realized that we were traversing the side of a snowy, slippery mountain, above the darkest and, therefore, deepest part of the lake. If Noah and I fell, there was no shore to land on, no shallow water to buffer our fall. Just a frigid black hole that would likely swallow us, especially because I had the weight of a toddler harnessed to my back. Even now, as I type these words so many years later, my fingers feel numb, my legs rigid, and my breath shallow. My heart is racing, my eyes are filling with tears, and there's a closing in my throat and tightness and bracing in my chest. Pure, primal terror.

In Somatic Experiencing, you would recognize this as a freeze or shock response.

In that moment on the mountain, everything slowed to a screeching halt, as if my body and mind were preparing for a head-on collision. I couldn't talk, move, think, or act. I felt completely paralyzed. Like a deer caught in headlights, I was as frozen as the glaciers above us. As I stood there, stunned, I couldn't peel my eyes away from the dark mass of water fifty yards below us. I knew I needed to move, but my limbs were locked in place. Having enough clarity to recognize that I had little control of my body and balance, I decided it would be safer if we weren't standing. I slowly lowered my body to the ground, leaning back and to one side so Noah's carrier wedged into the snow.

"Are you okay?" I heard. I hadn't realized a line of hikers had gathered behind us. Like a line of cars taking their turn on a single lane road, people were making their way one by one across this steep ledge.

I tried to speak, but nothing came out. I couldn't talk.

"Do you need help? Hey, I think they need help!" a hiker shouted to David.

David. In my distress, I had forgotten David was there. Thank God he was! The most microscopic of sighs escaped from my lips as I was able to shift my eyes slowly ahead, making eye contact with my husband.

"Honey, stay where you are. I'm coming," he said calmly.

Tears began to well over, falling onto my checks. I inhaled sharply, as if I were coming up for air for the first time. I was starting to feel more present. Words came back to me as helplessness abated.

"Noah, baby, Mama's got you. Daddy's coming, baby," I assured my son. "David, I'm stuck. I'm frozen, and I can't move," I said matter-of-factly. By this point, David was just a few steps away.

The coiled muscles in my limbs began to release and collapse. I felt as though I was floating above my body, observing the scene below. Dissociation took over.

Dissociation (leaving the present either through the body or mind) is common when your nervous system becomes overwhelmed.

The next thing I knew, David was next to me, holding my hand. The physical contact granted me an unobstructed path back to the present. As my eyes took in his face, I instinctually reached my hand back over my shoulder to interlock Noah's little fingers in mine. That instantly helped me feel more present, and I could feel my body thawing as I went from numb nothingness to the beginning waves of trembling and shaking.

My body and nervous system weren't shaking because of the cold. This was different. This was the adrenaline and cortisol of my flight response, signaling that it was time to mobilize and get the hell out of there.

Within minutes, David and another hiker slowly hoisted me up. As I gathered my footing, I knew that if I allowed them to carry us off that mountainside, the adrenaline and cortisol could remain stuck in my body, creating a toxic internal environment. I knew this was the moment that would dictate whether this would be another traumatic moment for my nervous system or a moment of resilience and completion. I knew my nervous system needed to see this overwhelming experience through, and that no one could do that for me, while also recognizing I couldn't do it alone.

"I can walk. I need to walk," I stated directly. "But I also need your support for balance." We slowly shuffled back to the tree line, and with each pressing step, I leaned into the jolt of energy in my limbs as well as the roaring heat that now radiated from within.

I tracked the internal mobilization in my body, knowing it was doing exactly what it knew how to do best—keep me alive.

Just like that mother moose fighting to protect her own babies.

As soon as my right foot crossed the threshold back into the forest and the cover of trees, I let out a loud, spontaneous sigh. "Do you need to sit down?" David asked as I brought my awareness back to my still-trembling limbs and racing heart. "No, no. I need to move out the rest of this energy," I replied as I began removing Noah from my back so David could carry him. We swiftly started to backtrack, and I saw an open area of brush and made my way to it.

"I need a few minutes to get this out," I repeated.

My nervous system had gone from a freeze state to now thawing out in a flight response with still more survival energy to express and discharge.

As I stood in the open brush, I began to slowly shake my hands as if I'd just washed them. My fingertips tingled as my arms joined in, followed next by my feet and then my legs. Shaking, tingling, sweating, grunting, and vocalizing, the primal response of my nervous system was being expelled from each inch of my body.

Doing this is one of the crucial five steps of Somatic Experiencing that you'll read about in part II.

It didn't take long for the waves of intensity to soften. Before I knew it, I was bent forward with one hand on my knee and the other instinctively reaching out for David. As he took my hand in his, my nervous system landed back into regulation. Back into safety, connection, and rest and digest. Slowly standing up straight, I brought awareness to my center of gravity, to my balance, and to the sturdiness of my feet. I took one tiny step forward with my right foot and gently leaned my weight onto it, as if walking on ice and carefully testing its solidity. I stepped horizontally to my immediate right and did the same on my left side.

Knowing that dissociation can linger long after an experience, I was intentional about grounding back into my body as best I could.

Now able to look back out at Lake Josephine with peace and clarity, I knew the stress response cycle had completed.

Fast-forward to the present. As I sit here now in our library, I look across the room to the framed photo of Noah sitting on the blue shore of Lake Josephine taken just a short time after my moments of terror. Even now, remembering that I eventually found safety and peace in the aftermath of the event, I can feel a sigh of relief and a settling in my body.

Thanks to my intentional slowing down and somatic processing on that mountainside, I was able to return to that very same trail four months later with my mother. The glacier snow had melted by then, and I no longer felt paralyzed or even fazed when hiking there.

By allowing the experience to complete, by understanding and riding the natural waves of my nervous system, I can now look back on what happened with appreciation for the ways in which my body instinctively went into survival mode and helped me through it.

Let's now take a look at how the body's nervous system works, and why, and ways you can harness its innate power through Somatic Experiencing.

Understanding Your Nervous System

Your nervous system informs nearly every aspect of your life and well-being—your thoughts, behaviors, emotions, sensations, hormones, muscular system, viscera, fascia, immune system, impulses, and more. It supports four main functions:

1. Voluntary and involuntary movement

2. Maintaining your body's internal homeostasis by overseeing and supporting many of your body's automatic functions, like your heart rate, digestion, metabolism, body temperature, hormones, stress and survival responses, respiration, tissue repair, sleep-wake cycle, and more

3. Acting as your internal surveillance system, sensing and responding to stimuli and perceived threats and initiating the release of hormones to manage your stress and survival responses

4. Processing your thoughts, feelings, and emotions

The Polyvagal Theory

The Polyvagal Theory (PVT) is a breakthrough framework for understanding how the nervous system operates. Originated by psychologist and neuroscientist Dr. Stephen Porges, PVT highlights the nervous system's role in our *safety, connection,* and *regulation.* Porges believes that when humans feel safe, their nervous systems support the homeostatic functions of health, growth, and restoration, while simultaneously becoming more accessible for connection to other humans. Porges first introduced PVT during his presidential address at the annual meeting of the Society for Psychophysiological Research in 1994. His colleague, medical therapist Deb Dana, translated PVT into a working therapeutic model, and together they founded the Polyvagal Institute, which trains medical professionals (including myself). Today, PVT provides a supporting foundation for many therapy modalities, including Somatic Experiencing. What you'll read next will highlight the teachings, practices, and applications of PVT, as developed by Porges and Dana.

PVT has three organizing principles:

1. **Co-regulation:** Our nervous system prioritizes connection to others as a means of survival.

2. **Neuroception, or "detection without awareness":** Our body has an internal surveillance system that monitors or senses for cues of safety or danger, outside our mind's awareness. In other words, it takes place in our subconscious.

3. **Hierarchy:** Our nervous system follows a predictable pathway for survival when faced with perceived threat.

This chapter will explore each principle in depth.

Co-Regulation: The Science of Connection

Co-regulation is the science of togetherness that proves that we truly are *better together*. Humans enter the world hardwired for connection, making it a biological imperative—it's something we need to survive. Not only do we rely on our caregivers to nourish us, put a roof over our head, keep us safe, and tend to us, but on a nervous system level, our ability to be soothed and comforted by others dictates our ability to be soothed and comforted by ourselves later. From the moment we're born, we begin the lifelong and wordless experience of subconsciously seeking connection and togetherness with other nervous systems.

I experienced this firsthand when my children were born. Although

I had read research about these instincts, I was overwhelmed with pure love when both of my babies sought out moments for bonding and connection, even immediately after birth. They both looked for my face upon entering the world and did the "breast crawl" within minutes of being born, which is when a newborn army-crawls toward their mother's breast during skin-to-skin contact without external interference.

In the days and weeks after their birth, I was fascinated by my children's seemingly superhero-like senses that alerted them when I was near or far. "It's because they have an acute sense of smell for your breast milk, which they need for survival," my pediatrician once told me. But I also knew that they could accurately sense and attune themselves to my presence because of "heart coherence." The science of heart coherence suggests that the heart's magnetic field is the strongest rhythmic field produced by the human body. Extending several feet into the space around us, it carries important information about our emotional, physical, and energetic state. When you are around another person long enough, your heart rate will start to match theirs, making connection both a regulating resource and a cause for dysregulation, if you are around someone who's anxious, angry, or depressed.

I witnessed the impact of heart coherence in the way my babies would suddenly wake and fuss or cry when I'd leave the room. Or how their breath slowed and their sleep deepened when they were in my arms or lying skin-to-skin on my chest—a bonding experience my midwives had encouraged me to do as much as possible. Or how they'd match my moments of overwhelm and overstimulation with tears of their own.

Because of PVT, I knew that these first few years of their life would lay the foundation for much of their nervous system's development and that my own nervous system health played a large role in that, thanks to co-regulation. I knew that throughout their formative years, until it was ready to stand on its own, their nervous system would mirror the state of my nervous system, a concept known as "mirror neurons" or "mirror emotions." If I was anxious, they would be anxious. If I was depressed, they would feel depressed. If I felt calm, they would experience calm.

Starting in infancy, healthy moments of connection with others allows our underdeveloped nervous systems to be supported and regulated, while moments of disconnection or the need for protection from others increases our overwhelm and reinforces habitual survival patterns that we carry into adulthood. In a world that prioritizes independence, we often assume that our ability to self-soothe is developed before we acquire the ability to be soothed by others. Yet PVT shows the opposite to be true: it's co-regulation that creates the foundation upon which we learn to self-regulate. Because our nervous system is hardwired to prioritize connection, if we do not have healthy connection in our developmental years, we may grow up to learn that because we can't feel safe with others, we therefore cannot feel safe by ourselves. As Porges says: "Trauma compromises our ability to engage with others by replacing patterns of connection with patterns of protection."

The Social Engagement System

Porges explains that we have a complex social engagement system built into our neuroanatomy through the connection via our vagus nerve between our heart and face. The vagus nerve communicates the state of our parasympathetic nervous system, so our face truly shows what our heart is feeling. The social engagement system is always sending or seeking out signals of welcome or of warning through our eyes, ears, voice, facial expressions, and head movement. Likewise, it searches for the same kinds of signals from those around us and takes in that information.

When I made eye contact with David on our hike, I felt a surge of safety in my system. His calm voice from across the trail, the touch of his hand, and holding little Noah's fingers in mine—these were profound moments that brought comfort and regulation when my system was too overwhelmed to self-regulate on its own.

Another example of our social engagement system at work is when we instinctively use baby talk, coos, and terms of endearment when communicating with a baby (or a puppy) without even thinking about it. PVT explains that when we're in a regulated state, the vagus nerve sends signals to our larynx and pharynx that initiate increased porosity of our vocal cords—the rhythmic variation or up-and-down intonation of our voice. It's this increased porosity that creates a deeper experience of co-regulation. This is just another example highlighting that, more than anything, your nervous system is always going to prioritize connection.

The social engagement system is comprised of connected pathways along the vagus nerve and the nerves in our face and head. It controls all of the following:

1. **Our facial expression (emotional expression):** When we are in a state of regulation and connection, we have full access to emotional expression and send clear, welcoming messages. As we move into states of protection or disconnection, we lose access to facial expression.

2. **Our eyelids (social gaze):** When we are in a state of regulation and connection, we have kind and present eyes. As we move into states of protection or disconnection, our pupils dilate to scan for threat or become distant and gaze downward as we go into shutdown.

3. **Our middle ear (hears human voices):** When we are in a state of regulation and connection, our middle ear muscles activate to hear mid-range frequencies, or human voices, leading to more meaningful conversation. As we move into states of protection or disconnection, we have mid-range hearing loss as our lower

ear muscles become activated to listen to low-frequency sounds, or evolutionarily speaking—sounds of threat-like growls, thuds, and bangs. This is why it's hard to have conversations when we're in states of survival.

4. **Our head turn and tilt (social gesture, orienting):** When we are in a state of regulation and connection, a gentle tilt of the head invites curiosity and connection with others. This turning of the neck stimulates the vagus nerve for regulation.

In a world where we're more connected through technology, social media, news, etc., yet more isolated and lonely than ever, connection is becoming harder to find. The high levels of dysregulation and mental illness we're seeing in young people today may be a result of the lack of the face-heart connection and authentic co-regulation.

It's also important to note that just as we can co-regulate with people to help us feel safe, people also can dysregulate us through co-regulation. If you're constantly around someone who is anxious all the time, your nervous system is going to experience more anxiety. If you're around someone who's depressed all the time, your system might start to take on symptoms of depression as well.

Neuroception: The Science of Safety

"Neuroception" is your body's ability to detect threats and safety, far below your conscious control, without your mind's awareness. In other words, it's physical awareness that comes without *perception*. Stephen Porges coined the term *neuroception* to describe the way our autonomic nervous system perceives cues of safety or danger without involving the thinking parts of the brain.

The thought-free process of neuroception begins in the brain stem, otherwise known as the reptilian brain, which governs survival instincts and impulses and carries the language of the senses. When thinking about this oldest and most primitive part of the brain, picture a lizard. A lizard takes in the world through the full use of its senses. It scans through sound, sight, smell, and touch. It pauses, orients, darts away, or freezes. We, too, have those same instinctual abilities to sense our environment and respond impulsively. For instance, many of our gut instincts and intuitions, like our ability to sense or feel when an environment or person's vibe is "off," are our Spidey Senses of neuroception.

Triggers and Glimmers

Porges discovered that the nervous system is always listening to what's going on in and around us to gauge whether we are safe or not safe. Through neuroception, the nervous system leans into three pathways of subconscious awareness: inside, outside, and between. This scanning takes place:

- *Inside* **your body:** Viscera, muscles, and organs
- *Outside* **in your external environment:** Both the immediate world around you and the larger world
- *Between* **you and other people:** On a nervous system level, not a brain level

When a neuroceptive cue of safety is present, we call these your "glimmers." When a neuroceptive cue of danger is present (like the grizzlies my system was scanning for), we call these your "triggers." It's important to note that what feels safe and not safe is unique from person to person. The following table offers some possible examples.

	INSIDE	OUTSIDE	BETWEEN
Danger cues (triggers)	Heart racing, shortness of breath, brain fog, nausea, anxiety, overwhelm, anger, shame, fear	Loud noise, chaos, unsafe weather, world events, being alone, unfamiliarity, lack of food or shelter	Yelling, monotone voice, stiff face, being blamed, ignored, rejected, or judged

	INSIDE	OUTSIDE	BETWEEN
Safety cues (glimmers)	Calm heart, steady breath, clear mind, relaxed posture, peacefulness, excitement, control	Familiarity, sunshine, calm environment (sounds and smells), access to food and shelter	Smiling, welcoming vocal tone, kind eyes, acceptance, laughter, play, compassion

Based on the PVT framework, Porges and Dana developed the Polyvagal Triggers and Glimmers Map, which helps you identify what uniquely feels safe (your glimmers) and not safe (your triggers) for your nervous system. You can complete this map on page 272 in Appendix A.

The Triggered Brain

To explore what it really means to be "triggered," let's first review the brain science. More specifically, when it comes to triggers, much of the experience lives within the subconscious brain—the reptilian brain, or brain stem, and the mammalian brain, or limbic system. The limbic system is responsible for connection, emotion, and memory, and most importantly in relation to trauma, it contains the amygdala, or the "threat center" of the brain. Because the limbic system is closely connected to the brain stem/reptilian brain, it can influence the basic functions governed there, such as breathing, heartbeat, digestion, and more.

The amygdala itself has an incredibly important function: to protect us from perceived threats. When the amygdala receives a neuroceptive cue of danger (a trigger) from the reptilian brain (again, think of the lizard sensing the environment), then a cascade of survival responses follow:

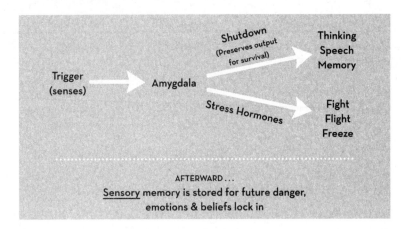

1. Your body releases stress hormones, like adrenaline and cortisol, to prepare you to mobilize—*like the adrenaline I was overwhelmed with on the mountain.*
2. This initiates your physiological impulse to fight, flight, or shut down—*like when I was going into panic mode yet couldn't move.*
3. When the amygdala is activated, nonessential areas of the brain shut down (including the thinking, talking, and remembering parts of the brain) so your brain can prioritize output for survival—*this is why I couldn't speak when the hikers asked if I needed help.*

There's a reason why, when the amygdala takes over, we react before we can even think. Areas of the brain that aren't necessary for survival become impaired or can go completely offline, including the Broca's area for speech, the prefrontal cortex for thinking, and the hippocampus for storing memory. In essence, in the pursuit of survival, the ancient and primal wisdom of the reptilian and mammalian brain will always override that of the newest (in evolutionary terms) human brain or neocortex. So when you're triggered, don't be surprised if logic, rationale, or problem-solving skills go out the window.

We also often react before we can think when we're triggered because the amygdala literally responds faster than the thinking brain, sending messages from the brain to the body in 200 milliseconds, versus the prefrontal cortex, which sends messages down to the body in three to five seconds. This is why we impulsively *react* without pause. Like when we drop a knife or a pair of scissors, we don't contemplate what to do but instead instinctually kick our foot back so the sharp object doesn't harm us.

Sometimes we look at our reactions and berate ourselves when they seem completely incongruent or irrational given the reality of the situation. "Why did I do that?!" we might ask ourselves when we run away, freak out, or explode, without realizing that our conscious/rational thoughts never stood a chance against the instincts and impulse of the subconscious/irrational brain. Now, this doesn't *excuse* harmful or destructive behavior, but it certainly *explains* it. However, the good news is, we can change our default reactions through intentionally and proactively practicing new responses, creating new neural pathways and procedural patterns or impulses of the nervous system.

LISA'S STORY

A client named Lisa had spent years suffering from relentless insomnia before coming to work with me. She had tried all the medications, remedies, and relaxation practices—all with no long-term relief. After seeing countless sleep specialists who couldn't give her a diagnosis or answer, she chalked it up to years of stress and the effects of allostatic load (the cumulative wear and tear on the body due to chronic stress). So she cut back on her hours at work, committed to a healthier diet that would fuel her, scheduled family trips, and tried to *take it easy.* Unfortunately, the insomnia wouldn't let up.

It didn't take long after working together for us to find that the stress that was keeping Lisa awake at night wasn't a reflection of her present-day pressures, but instead was a subconscious association of fear of the dark, or more specifically, fear of what darkness had brought in her younger years, when she was repeatedly assaulted by a family member. Lisa couldn't believe it. "But that doesn't make any rational sense!" she said. "I'm not afraid of the dark!" Yet her body showed us a different story.

When I worked with Lisa in a session to *rehearse* her nightly routine through visualization, her body showed us, quite clearly, that the moment Lisa shut off the lights, there would be activation. Her shoulders would tense, her breath would go shallow, and she'd experience dissociation or numbness in the lower part of her body. This had become Lisa's normal; it had been all she'd known for so long, which is why she perhaps couldn't consciously recognize that every night as the lights went out, her body and physiology were stuck in the past, reliving the survival responses of those moments over and over.

Through our work together, Lisa was able to restore a sense of presence and safety in her body, allowing her to finally somatically process that experience with agency and empowerment. The stress and survival hormones from the past were finally expelled. Over time, Lisa's trigger to the dark became less intense, along with the insomnia.

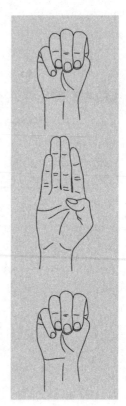

FLIPPING YOUR LID

Dr. Dan Siegel, renowned clinical professor of psychiatry at the University of California, Los Angeles, School of Medicine, pioneered a concept called "Flipping Your Lid," in which we can use our hand to show what happens to our brain when we're triggered. In this model, our fingers are our upstairs brain (neocortex), and our thumb (amygdala), palm (mammalian brain), and wrist (reptilian brain) are our downstairs brain. Flipping Your Lid explains:

1. The brain works best when the upstairs (thinking) and downstairs (emotional) brains work together.

2. When we're triggered, our upstairs thinking brain flips up and our downstairs emotional brain is in charge. This means it's hard for our upstairs brain to help our downstairs brain stay calm— that is, we become "irrational."

3. When we "flip our lid," we need to get our upstairs and downstairs brains collaborating again so our upstairs brain can support our downstairs brain. This means we first have to calm our emotions and impulses throughout the body, before the thinking/rational brain can come back online.

A Dysregulated "Security System"

When we're triggered by situations that evoke past hurt, we can think of it like a smoke signal from the past. The signal is present, but there may not be an actual fire. And when we experience this trigger, we likely will have the same physical and mental reactions as we had to the original trauma. It's as if our subconscious is screaming, "We're in danger *now*!" when it really means, "We were in danger *then*."

Again, think of your nervous system as your built-in security system. It's always alert, scanning quietly in the background as you go about your day, ready to protect you from any perceived threat. When a perceived threat is present, whether real threat or not—a dog barking, a loud noise, a baby crying, your boss yelling, a black hole of deep water below you as you hike on a mountainside—your nervous system responds. And when you've already survived or witnessed a threat, your nervous system takes on an additional role. It's not just going to detect and protect you from seemingly normal triggers, but it also will do its utmost to prevent whatever trauma that happened in the past from happening again in the present.

Think of it this way: If burglars broke into your home through your windows, you'd need a security system that didn't just monitor the doors, but also monitored the windows. Your need for protection has been heightened. Likewise, you can have a security system that is faulty if you have trauma that is *unhealed*. It may sound an alarm 24/7, even when a threat is no longer present. Or it may not sound an alarm at all, even when a real threat is present—a clear neuroceptive mismatch. This is what we'd call a "dysregulated" nervous system, one that's stuck in chronic states of survival.

Same Equals Safe

There's what we *know* to be safe, and then there's what the nervous system *feels* is safe. And more often than not, these two things look very different. It's important to note that your nervous system will always prioritize what feels *familiar*, even if it's not good for you. According to your physiology, same equals safe because it's predictable. Your nervous system doesn't *think*, so it can't conceptualize or rationalize what is and isn't safe (like the abusive relationship, the toxic work environment, or the procrastination that's putting your job at risk).

More than anything, your nervous system wants to follow a predictable path of familiarity. We often see these patterns of being stuck in the same dysfunctional cycles as self-sabotage, but this is merely your nervous system following the same pathways of self-protection that have served you until now. The reality is, your nervous system doesn't even know how to sabotage you. It merely gravitates to what it's already known, experienced, and survived. Over time, continually giving your nervous system small and tolerable—what we call titrated—moments of "real safety" will create a new collection of *familiar evidence* your system needs to know that change is possible.

Hierarchy: Science of Regulation

The third organizing principle of PVT is that the nervous system works in a hierarchy that prioritizes safety and connection. This means your body's and your nervous system's responses are going to follow a predictable path.

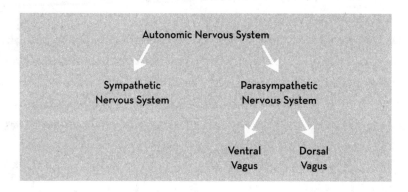

The autonomic nervous system is comprised of two branches, the parasympathetic nervous system (PNS) and the sympathetic nervous system (SNS), and it responds to our experiences via a hierarchy of three predictable pathways: the ventral vagal complex, the sympathetic nervous system, and the dorsal vagal complex.

The Parasympathetic Nervous System

The PNS has two pathways, which are located in the vagus nerve:

1. **The ventral vagal pathway:** This is your *rest and digest state*. When you are in this state, your system promotes and prioritizes feelings of safety and connection (to others, to yourself, and to the world). You feel at ease in your body, empowered to manage whatever stress comes your way, and engaged with the world around you.

2. **The dorsal vagal pathway:** This is your *shutdown or collapsed state*. When extreme danger arises and you cannot fight or flee, the ancient and oldest dorsal nervous system takes over and you revert to your evolutionary beginnings of immobilization (think hibernation) as a means to survive. When buried under extreme threat or overwhelm, dorsal disconnects you from yourself, from others, and from the world around you. In this state, you feel numb, not here, and a sense of nothingness.

The Sympathetic Nervous System

The SNS houses your fight-or-flight responses and is found in both the spinal and peripheral nerves. The sympathetic branch mobilizes you for action and regulates the stress hormones adrenaline and cortisol (arousal) as it prepares you to either protect, play, or perform. It's most active when you're alert, excited, engaged in physical activities, or confronted with an emergency or threat.

You can think of your nervous system like a car, in which the PNS is the brake pedal and the SNS is the gas pedal:

- When you are in a ventral state, the brake pedal allows you to gently slow down, unwind, and connect to the present.

- When you are in a sympathetic state, the gas pedal mobilizes you to give you the energy to take action.

- When you are in a dorsal state, an *emergency* brake pedal initiates when the gas pedal of your sympathetic fight-or-flight response is too overwhelming.

Historically, the nervous system was believed to include just two distinct branches, parasympathetic rest and digest, and sympathetic fight or flight. However, PVT illustrates that the parasympathetic nervous system is further organized into its own two separate pathways, as I explained above. This remarkable discovery changes the way we previously understood the landscape of our nervous system. Instead of having two states, we have three, ventral, sympathetic, and dorsal. Stephen Porges dedicated much of his research to the exploration of these two new vagal pathways—the term *vagal* in PVT refers to the vagus nerve, and *poly* simply means "more than one," or ventral and dorsal. These branches start from different parts of the brain stem. The ventral pathway emerges from the front of the body, and the dorsal pathway from the back of the body.

The ventral vagus governs the parts of the body above the diaphragm, as it connects to our lungs, throat, and heart. It also influences facial expressions, speech rhythms, and our sense of surroundings. (Again, think of the face-heart connection in our social engagement system that promotes connection when we're in ventral.) This branch helps regulate our heart rate and blood pressure and supports feelings of safety, communication, and learning. Via the ventral vagus we have access to our neocortex or rational brain, where thinking, learning, and talking happen.

The dorsal vagus, located along the back of the body, predominantly governs the organs below the diaphragm, as it connects to the stomach, liver, kidneys, spleen, colon, and intestines and oversees digestive function. The dorsal state can be thought of as our body's immobilization and conservation system—during danger, it redirects blood away from our limbs and inward to our vital organs, slowing down our heart rate and breath. We can experience this response as fainting, dissociating, and/or collapsing in the face of life-threatening situations. We also can feel its effects in milder forms, like social withdrawal or emotional numbness.

Eric and the Autonomic Loop

Eric came to me in a season of extreme burnout. At the time he was taking a sabbatical from work, having handed over the reins of his multiple global companies to one of his business associates. This wasn't the first time Eric had needed a break, exhausted and running on fumes. This was a cycle, a pattern that had begun in his high school years. He'd excel, overachieve, and overperform and then he'd crash, collapsing deeper into shutdown each time.

It's a pattern I see often with my *high-performing* clients, the ones whose résumés, accolades, and professional titles stand out among the rest. The obsession and pressure to perform—whether that be inherited, or as a means of escape, or they believe a reflection of their worth—consumes them. They work, work, work, keeping the foot on the gas as they chronically live in the sympathetic state of productivity and mobilization . . . until one day, when the gas runs out and they end up in dorsal and burnout—the state of conservation, rest, and repair. And because they've now created work conditions that require *all of* themselves, or because they don't know how to pace themselves, they eventually fall back into the same vicious pattern. This is what Porges and Dana refer to as an "autonomic loop," or a frequent cycle between two states.

After working with Eric to somatically heal this subconscious pattern in his nervous system—which we found dated back to childhood, where he equated performance with love as his emotionally distant father gave him attention and praise only when he'd do well—he was able to create more sustainable boundaries around work output. He finally found himself in a place where he no longer sought out external praise and instead was motivated by his own internal and intrinsic value.

THE AUTONOMIC TIMELINE

Just like the brain, the nervous system has developed through millions of years of evolution, adapting and building upon itself over time to meet our basic needs for survival. Stephen Porges calls this the autonomic timeline. In evolutionary terms, the dorsal parasympathetic pathway is the most ancient branch of the autonomic nervous system, found in all primitive vertebrates dating back 500 million years, while the sympathetic nervous system emerged 400 million years ago with the evolution of reptiles. Ventral is the most recent pathway. It evolved 200 million years ago and gave rise to our social engagement system and our ability to find safety in communication and connection.

Hierarchy: The Polyvagal Ladder

To demonstrate the predictable path or hierarchy that the nervous system follows throughout the day and in response to safety and danger, Porges created a useful tool called the Polyvagal Ladder. The Body-First Healing Roadmap will guide you in mapping out your own Polyvagal Ladder, which will give you a deeper understanding of your own unique nervous system.

How the Polyvagal Ladder Works

Every day, you move up and down the nervous system ladder—your own unique Polyvagal Ladder. Imagine the following while looking at the illustration below:

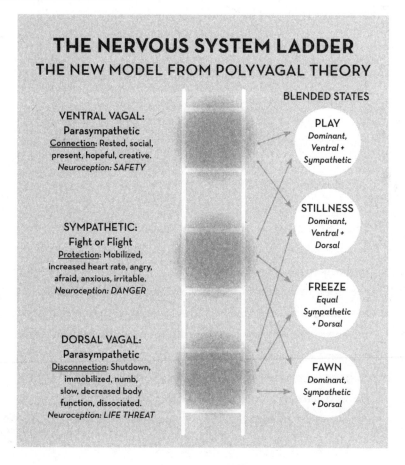

- You wake up on the "right side of the bed," or in a ventral state. Here, at the top of the ladder, you feel safe enough to connect with your internal world, the external environment, and those around you.

- Now imagine that as you stand on that ladder, you're also wearing an empty backpack. Throughout the day, as you experience more stressors, triggers, or neuroceptive cues of danger, weights will be added to your backpack. Naturally, as the stressors or triggers pile on, you begin to come down the ladder due to the weight pulling you down. According to the built-in hierarchy of your nervous system, the first predictable response you will have is to fight or flee via the sympathetic branch.

- If fighting or fleeing does not bring you out of that perception of danger, or if it's not an option—for instance, some children grow up in environments where fighting back is going to create more danger or running away means there's not going to be a roof over their heads—then your nervous system will naturally pull you down into your dorsal response of immobilization and shutdown.

- You now may be wondering how to get back up to the top. Just as there's a predictable hierarchy going down, the same order remains in place when you move up. In other words, if you're at the bottom of the ladder in dorsal, you can't simply Spider-Man your way back up to ventral (although that would be nice). When we are in a state of shutdown, we still carry the adrenaline and cortisol released when the sympathetic response of fight or flight/mobilization began. So to move up and through the sympathetic state on the path to a ventral state, we must discharge or release those pent-up survival hormones. See Appendix A to learn exactly how to do this.

Common Characteristics of the Polyvagal Ladder

TOP OF THE LADDER	EMOTIONAL STATE	KEY WORD
State: Ventral vagal	Safe and connected	Connection

- What you say: I am okay. The world is welcoming and filled with opportunity.

MIDDLE OF THE LADDER	EMOTIONAL STATE	KEY WORD
State: Sympathetic	Angry or anxious	Protection

- What you say: I am crazy. I am toxic. The world is unfriendly, scary, and exploding.

BOTTOM OF THE LADDER	EMOTIONAL STATE	KEY WORD
State: Dorsal vagal	Shutdown	Disconnection

- What you say: I am unlovable, invisible, lost, and alone. The world is cold, empty, and uninhabitable.

The harrowing hiking experience I had in Montana beautifully illustrates the nervous system's brilliant and innate ability to keep us safe. After the initial moment of extreme threat and the pure terror that followed, my system was able to bring me into a state of shutdown. Then, the co-regulation I was able to experience with my husband and son pulled me up the ladder toward a ventral state. My muscles then trembled and shook to discharge all the stuck adrenaline and cortisol flooding my body. Each moment had waves of activation that I rode in order to climb back into a safe, connected, and regulated state.

We Can't Always Be in a Ventral State

There's a common misconception that the goal of nervous system regulation is to stay at the top of the ladder in ventral 24/7. However, the average human with a healthy and regulated nervous system goes up and down the Polyvagal Ladder nearly one hundred times every day! This is what we call a "flexible," resilient, or regulated nervous system—one that can move up and down the ladder with ease, without getting *stuck*. In contrast, a nervous system that isn't flexible or that lives in a constant state of sympathetic or dorsal is what we consider a "rigid" or dysregulated nervous system.

Blended States in the Polyvagal Ladder

In addition to the three nervous system states, Porges also argued that we have *blended* states, which include play, stillness, and freeze and fawn. As illustrated in the Polyvagal Ladder image on page 95, in blended moments, your nervous system experiences more than one physiological response at one time.

Play

In moments of play, you are in both a ventral and a sympathetic state. You utilize the mobilizing energy and adrenaline of your sympathetic fight-or-flight response when you're moving with intention during any kind of workout, sports activity, or dance, or when you just play in general (like going to the playground with your kids, for instance). And although you're in a physical fight-or-flight response, because there are no neuroceptive cues of danger, you aren't experiencing the emotional response of anger or anxiety. Instead, you receive cues of safety so you are emotionally anchored in your parasympathetic ventral state, where you feel connected, happy, adventurous, and excited.

Fawning

Fawning, commonly referred to as appeasing or people-pleasing, is not its own nervous system state, even though many people assume it is. Fawn is a specific blended response of the sympathetic flight state and the dorsal shutdown state. When we fawn, we're disconnecting and shutting down the parts of ourselves that we want to be heard— our dorsal state. In this regard, we avoid confrontation, advocate for our own wants and needs, and set boundaries. We tend toward avoidance from an emotional response of fear (flight response)—we're worried, anxious, and/or afraid that setting the boundary, advocating for ourselves, or confronting the person will lead to rejection, abandonment, judgment, further harm, etc. So instead, we tend to others and put their wants and needs before our own to diffuse potential additional danger.

Freeze

Freeze is a blended response of extreme sympathetic fight or flight and dorsal shutdown. We commonly refer to freeze as having one foot on the gas (sympathetic) and one foot on the brake (dorsal) at the same time. Freeze occurs in moments of life threat, shock, or horror, when our system becomes so overwhelmed by the charge of sympathetic hormones that we have an immediate deer-in-the-headlights response. We feel mobilized but in shock and unable to move.

FREEZE	SHUTDOWN/COLLAPSE
Muscles & spine stiffen and tense	Muscles & spine collapse and go limp
Increased: heart rate, blood pressure	Decreased: heart rate, blood pressure, temperature
Eyes widen, hyperaware, feeling panic, overwhelm, terror, or life threat	Blank stare, feeling dissociated or detached from body, mind & present
Deer in the headlights: full of mobilizing energy, but can't release it (immobilized)	Like a limp animal, fainting or playing dead, we feel slow, tired, and immobilized
State of stuckness, bracing for impact, but ready to fight or flee	State of nothingness, hopelessness, no pain and numbness, withdrawal & energy conservation

It's important to differentiate between a freeze response and dorsal shutdown. We've long thought of the nervous system's possible responses to a perceived threat as fight, flight, or freeze. However, PVT argues that the actual possible responses we experience are fight, flight, or shutdown. And although our freeze and shutdown responses may appear similar, they actually differ quite a bit, as shown in the illustration. These two responses can feel and look differently *within* the brain, body, and nervous system, but they often can resemble each other behaviorally. Behaviors include isolating, procrastinating, spacing out, bingeing TV, and dissociating.

Functional Freeze

To add one more blended state to the mix, it's important to mention functional freeze, which can be considered the state of "autopilot." Freeze is also a blended response of sympathetic fight or flight and dorsal shutdown. Rather than shock, functional freeze is a mobilizing state of shutdown. In this state, we function throughout the day, yet are detached from our body, our emotions, and our internal landscape. We seem "normal" on the outside, yet we are suffering on the inside. It can seem like we are *going through the motions* yet lack emotion. Or we may muscle or power through or appear unfazed. Our culture applauds putting on a brave face and completely detaching from our somatic experience, and it's safe to say that many of us struggle with this blended response. It is one of the five stuck personalities we will explore later in this book.

It can be really confusing when you start to come out of states of shutdown, freeze, and functional freeze, because now everything that's been numbed or suppressed comes to the surface. It can make people think that they're regressing. *Why am I feeling so much anxiety now? Why are these sensations coming up?* They criticize themselves without recognizing that this is a sign of progress, a sign of "thawing out" and moving up the ladder into fight or flight, where the nervous system once felt too overwhelmed to function.

The Link between Polyvagal Theory and Somatic Experiencing

PVT offers a clear path to regulation, one built on safety, connection, and the ability to discharge the stuck and stored survival charge by following the predictable path laid out in the nervous system's hierarchy. Porges (who is a longtime friend of Peter Levine) and PVT support Levine's original research. Unlike animals in the wild that can "shake" their bodies to eliminate stress and fear, humans often lack the ability to move through their stress response cycle. As a result, the residual fight-or-flight energy becomes "trapped" within the body. And when left untreated or unresolved, these overwhelming experiences in the nervous system can cause dysregulation, where we constantly feel triggered, even in the absence of real threat. Humans, of course, are much more complex creatures, so a simple shaking won't resolve our trauma.

Instead, Levine's framework of Somatic Experiencing focuses on regulating our nervous system by first building a foundation of safety. These are our resources, according to Somatic Experiencing, or glimmers, according to PVT. Our ability to create a felt sense of safety—inside and outside our bodies as well as between ourselves and others—promotes regulation and pulls us up the Polyvagal Ladder. After safety is established, the slow and gentle process of expressing or discharging what's still stuck and stored in the body begins, whether that's anger, fear, grief, or any other emotion. When we give the nervous system the opportunity to express what it couldn't in the past, it naturally comes back up the ladder to the ventral state of safety and connection.

What's more, in the process of creating more capacity to move through the pain of the past, we're creating a more flexible and resilient nervous system that can face everyday stress and triggers with more ease, now and in the future.

CHAPTER 6

How Your Childhood Attachment Informs Your Adult Relationships

We're just here to be memories for our kids. Once you're a parent, you're the ghost of your children's future.
—Matthew McConaughey, *Interstellar*

B ut my childhood was normal," clients would say. "I *know* my parents loved me." I've heard this too often in my time as a somatic practitioner, and truthfully, I used to voice this thought as well.

My response is almost always the same: "There's what we know, and there's what we feel. And sometimes, there's a mismatch between the two. For instance, although you can know through cognition that your parents loved you, did you also *feel*, back then, that they loved you?"

How often do we look back at our childhood with rose-colored glasses, rationalizing all the ways we were cared for, loved, and accepted? And although that may be true—although there may have been a roof over our head, food on the table, and no threat of violence and we think we "turned out normal"—it's important to remember that two things can be true at once. Our perception of having a seemingly ordinary childhood can coexist with the reality that there also could have been times when we *felt* unsafe, especially in our earliest years before we could even speak. Perhaps we encountered insufficient bonding and attunement from loving caregivers; or we had inadequate shielding from harmful circumstances or individuals; or we were raised in an atmosphere of abandonment, neglect, chaos, or fear.

This is the nature of attachment, or early relational wounds. The wounds that haunt us the most are often the ones hidden in plain sight. Attachment wounds can be covert; they don't always scream in your face. Instead, these wounds shape your instinctual choices, reactions, and feelings, creating potentially unloving and unhealthy learned beliefs and behaviors that show up in your life today. These are the impulses and reactions that echo the voice of the hurt child who still rules over your nervous system today and who, at every turn, will override your adult rational mind in moments of distress. We resort to our childlike selves in the ways we pull away from others, the ways we chase after relationships, or the ways we explode. And then, we shame and ridicule ourselves for our "irrational" behavior without recognizing that these are invaluable moments of opportunity—when these younger parts of us can finally experience the safety, attunement, and soothing they lacked in our formative years.

As Peter Levine famously says, "It's never too late to give yourself the childhood you deserve."

This chapter will help you explore that unique path back to yourself. Through acceptance and self-attunement, you'll create an *internal* sense (a feeling) that someone finally hears you, sees you, and has your back. From there, you'll begin to develop the innate capacity to set boundaries, walk with agency, and learn how to rise into your physiological power—which in turn will cultivate a healthier relationship to yourself, to others, and to the greater world around you.

The Origins of Attachment Theory

While working at a child's guidance clinic in the 1930s, John Bowlby, a renowned English psychiatrist who became known as the "father of attachment theory," explored the influence that a child's maternal bond (*attachment*) had on their social, emotional, and cognitive growth. At the time of his early research, prevailing Freudian theories attributed a child's behavior and development to internal driving factors like aggression, hunger, and sexuality while overlooking external influences. Bowlby challenged this notion as he observed emotionally troubled children in his care who had lacked early affection and experienced disrupted caregiving. Despite opposition, his work emphasized the significance of relational experiences in infancy and beyond.

It was through this clinical experience that Bowlby conceived his groundbreaking attachment theory, which provides the idea that our early bonds—our *attachments*—play a crucial role in lifelong functioning and development. He asserted that the primary caregiver, typically the mother, served as a vital "psychic organizer," essential for a child's successful cognitive, emotional, social, and behavioral development—and advocated for warm, consistent, and intimate relationships with caregivers for optimal health. He argued that attachment has four specific distinguishing characteristics:

- Proximity maintenance: Wanting to be near those to whom we are attached
- Safe haven: Being able to return to the caregiver for comfort and safety when faced with a fear or threat
- Secure base: The caregiver is the child's base, allowing them to explore safely
- Distress: Normal anxiety when the caregiver is absent

In addition to his human observations of mother-to-child bonding, Bowlby also was inspired by naturalistic observations of mammalian caregiving behaviors, highlighting striking parallels in survival instincts among various species. Notably, he observed in our primate relatives, chimpanzees and gorillas, that the young seek protection from an adult when frightened. This observation and many others led Bowlby to propose that humans, like their primate counterparts, are inherently wired to form deep emotional connections as a means of proximity, better ensuring our survival.

Expanding on the research, Mary Ainsworth, a psychologist and colleague of Bowlby's, developed the Strange Situation Classification (SSC) assessment method in 1969 to explore differences in attachment experiences among children. By first placing a child and mother in a strange room, she would observe the child's reaction to different circumstances, such as the mother leaving, strangers coming in and going, and more. Ainsworth's research revealed that as a result of these particular early mother-child interactions, predictable relational responses from the child would occur. She identified three primary attachment styles (relational patterns): secure, insecure-avoidant, and insecure ambivalent-resistant, all of which will be explored in this chapter. Subsequently, in 1986, a fourth attachment style, disorganized attachment, was identified by researchers Mary Main and Judith Solomon. Through this powerful science, we now know that the bonds we have with our caregivers likely will mirror the bonds we have in adulthood.

During the last eighty plus years, Bowlby's attachment theory has been extensively researched and established across various disciplines, including psychology, sociology, neuroscience, and developmental science. Tens of thousands of research papers, articles, books, and dissertations have been published on various aspects of attachment theory, covering concepts such as attachment styles, attachment behaviors, attachment-related disorders, and interventions. Many of these topics will be explored in this chapter, as we dive into our attachment histories and examine the role they play in our relationships and overall well-being today.

Attachment Basics

There are two lenses through which attachment is generally explored: our attachment in childhood, and our attachment styles in adulthood. Here, we'll explore both, starting first with attachment in childhood, recognizing that many of the personal and relational challenges we face in our adult lives today can be traced back to our earliest bonds.

Attachment is an emotional bond that forms in infancy and early childhood with our parent or caregiver. It plays a pivotal role in our childhood development and also influences our attachment patterns in adult relationships. Depending on the quality of this relationship, subconscious relational patterns (or attachment styles) become set in place, but are not entirely set in *stone*, by the time we are two years old. In fact, it's estimated that up to 80 percent of adults will have the same attachment style in adulthood as they had when they were eighteen months old. We see these predominant patterns in the ways we become either *secure* or *insecure* in our relationships with ourselves and others.

In the initial three years of life, known as the attachment phase, establishing a sense of safety and security with our primary caregivers is crucial. This foundation is essential for nurturing a healthy perception of self and the world, which in turn directly fosters healthy and meaningful adult relationships. Even more, nearly a century of research demonstrates that a secure attachment in childhood lays the groundwork for enduring mental and physical health later in life. The lifelong qualities we aspire for, such as strong relationships, resilience, and independence, are all rooted in attachment. Additionally, these early attachment experiences have a profound effect on the development of our nervous system, creating the blueprint for our ability to self-regulate and co-regulate.

Secure attachment to a caregiver provides three major benefits, including the following:

- Providing the child with a firm sense of safety and security
- Assisting the child in mastering emotional regulation by soothing distress, promoting joy, and supporting calm
- Offering a "secure base" from which to explore the world, promoting independence

The reverse holds true as well. A child who hasn't formed secure attachments with their caregivers may exhibit developmental disruptions, leading to learning struggles, emotional and behavioral challenges, and difficulty forming connections with others, that persist into adulthood. Fundamentally, secure attachment is intended to *protect* us from trauma, whereas an insecure attachment is *predictive* of trauma.

Attachment in Childhood

Circling back to the topic of co-regulation from the previous chapter, we must remember that connection to others is a biological imperative—a necessity for human survival—which is why our nervous system prioritizes connection through our social engagement system. Viewed through an evolutionary lens, fostering robust connections and preserving them offers both survival and reproductive benefits. Let's consider, for instance, the role that oxytocin (known as the "love hormone") plays in our lives. Oxytocin is responsible for facilitating milk flow from the breast ducts to the nipple, further nurturing the bond between mother and baby and also supporting nourishment. In addition, our bodies release oxytocin during moments of excitement with our intimate partner and during the experience of falling in love.

Science aside, you only need to get lost in a newborn's deep gaze to understand that humans are wired for connection. From birth, and even in utero, infants begin forming relationships with their caregivers and siblings. Renowned author David Wallin highlights in his book *Attachment in Psychotherapy* that babies start mirroring their parents' facial expressions only forty minutes after birth, underscoring the primal drive for connection. We make these biological bids for connection for a number of reasons, one being that it supports our development.

The nurturing gestures of parents, such as giving hugs, singing lullabies, and smiling, can offer lasting emotional and cognitive benefits to infants, potentially shielding them from heartbreak and adolescent challenges and even contributing to academic success later in life. The human brain, an awe-inspiring organ comprising more than 100 billion brain cells, exceeds the complexity of any known object in the universe—computers included. The most critical period for brain development begins in the womb and extends through the first year of life. By age three, a child's brain has attained nearly 90 percent of its adult size—with rapid brain growth and neural circuitry formation occurring at a remarkable rate of seven hundred to one thousand synapse connections per second. This is why the period of "infancy" extends to age three. So it should come as no surprise that interactions with caregivers during this time, when infants are facilitating the formation of millions of new connections, play a pivotal role in the brain's early wiring process. Through repeated interactions and communication, neural pathways are established, contributing to the development of implicit memories, impulses, beliefs, and cognitive abilities. It's safe to say that an infant's brain is both intricate and susceptible during this developmental phase.

In addition to cognitive development, secure attachment provides emotional support and regulation for a baby. For instance, when babies are born, they have an underdeveloped nervous system and brain. To regulate and soothe their intense reactions that are provoked by a stimulating world, their young nervous system relies entirely on their caregivers to bring them back to a physiological sense of safety and calm.

To really drive home this point, a longitudinal study conducted over thirty years by the Duke Global Health Institute found that a mother's affection in infancy predicts emotional distress in adulthood. In the study, which included 482 participants, researchers measured the level of affection a mother gave to her baby at eight months. The mental health, levels of anxiety and hostility, and general levels of distress of these babies was then assessed by researchers when they were grown adults (average age of thirty-four). The study revealed that babies whose mothers displayed the most "extravagant" affection toward them at the eight-month assessment grew into adults who exhibited notably reduced levels of distress, anxiety, and hostility. The strongest correlation was observed in the anxiety category. This trend persisted across all measurements, and the researchers concluded that the greater the mother's warmth, the less the child's distress in adulthood.

The vast collection of research on attachment theory not only challenges but disproves our cultural belief that when we give a child *too much attention*, we cripple them emotionally, raising a child who will grow up to be "clingy," "unstable," and "needy." Instead, the data highlights the exact opposite and demonstrates that we cannot love our children *too much* and that, in fact, the more you respond to your children, the more independent they become, because they believe there will always be a safe base from which to explore the world. As Gordon Neufeld, a Canadian developmental psychologist, says, "Attachment is the most significant dynamic in a child's life . . . and the purpose of attachment is to facilitate dependence."[1] Moreover, infants are instinctually wired to exhibit specific behaviors, known as "social releases," such as crying, smiling, and crawling, to foster closeness and contact with their mother or primary attachment figure. Ultimately, it's developmentally appropriate for babies and toddlers to show big emotions—to cry, to scream, and to use their bodies and power to get our attention—you know, those things labeled as "tantrums" or "meltdowns." If we make generalizations that babies should be "easy," we're setting standards for infants that don't line up with their biology. In fact, an "easy" or "good," quiet baby could be a troubling sign of an unhealthy internal detachment or dissociation.

In addition to its developmental benefits, attachment is also the base from which babies form their internal perception of themselves, which is constructed from the parents' responses and interactions with them. Because as children we perceive ourselves as our caregivers perceive us, when we're met with love and respect, we find that we can give that to ourselves more freely. This *secure base* promotes higher self-esteem, self-agency, confidence, independence, and the desire for exploration. Not only do we create beliefs about ourselves based on our parents' behaviors, but we also form expectations for future relational experiences based on our early attachments. For instance, consistent nurturing and attunement (understanding) from a parent will lead the child to expect similar treatment in other relationships. Conversely, if a parent yells or punishes using fear and threat, then the baby will anticipate the same in other relationships. Parents wield significant influence over their children's sense of self and others, creating inherent beliefs that either empower or stifle them throughout life.

As Alan Sroufe, a developmental psychologist at the Institute of Child Development at the University of Minnesota, explains, "Attachment is a relationship in the service of a baby's emotional regulation and exploration. It is the deep, abiding confidence a baby has in the availability and responsiveness of the caregiver."[2] Secure attachment reaps enormous benefits. According to the Minnesota Longitudinal Study of Parents and Children, a study aimed at looking at attachment patterns that started in 1975 and is ongoing, when a child senses a secure attachment with their caregiver, they will have the following:

- A greater sense of self-agency
- Better emotional regulation

- Higher self-esteem
- Better coping under stress
- More positive engagement in the preschool peer group
- Closer friendships in middle childhood
- Better coordination of friendships and social groups in adolescence
- More trusting, nonhostile romantic relationships in adulthood
- Greater social competence
- More leadership qualities
- Happier and better relationships with parents and siblings
- Greater trust in life

Perhaps you're wondering how an infant can begin to form such important beliefs about themselves and the world when their cognitive thinking and talking brain (the neocortex) hasn't even developed yet. Because we are inherently social beings, much of our communication relies on nonverbal cues such as body language, tone of voice, eye contact, and more. In our first year of life, we are living predominantly with our reptilian brain, or the brain stem, where the language we use to interpret the world around us is nonverbal and sensorial. This is how, as infants, we take in the cues of safety or danger from the world and individuals around us. Babies are especially receptive to these somatic cues, collecting a subconscious memory box of signals that are either welcoming or warning, which is stored as implicit (body) memory. These signals begin to create impulsive attachment patterns that we are likely to carry into adulthood. Examples of impulses might be avoiding eye contact if their caregiver's gaze is consistently full of rage, or suppressing emotion if it creates anxiety in the caregiver. Research shows that these biological "memories" that are laid down early alter our psychological and physiological systems later in life.

KRISTIN'S GAZE AVERSION

The eyes share our earliest stories in life. When I work with the eyes, I know I'm accessing patterns of attachment in my clients.

I could sense early on in our time together that Kristin had a history of attachment trauma. Her aversion to eye contact and consistent downward gaze during our sessions were initial signs.

Babies build reciprocity with others through eye contact by learning to first look at another's eyes, looking away, and looking back. This is also how they build entrainment (or how the baby learns to lead; i.e., *they choose* to look away and end the connection—developing the self) and affect synchrony (or emotional mirroring; i.e., when the adult smiles, the baby also smiles). When babies lack positive eye contact experiences, because of abuse or neglect, for instance, this relational contact of looking into someone else's eyes can become associated with fear or danger. The good news is that if harm was done, relational repair can be provided anytime throughout their life with another person.

By building a relational container with Kristin that felt safe, consistent, and connected, we were eventually able to lean into intentional eye work to build her capacity to receive people with her eyes, rather than pushing them away or avoiding them.

We explored boundary work, whereby Kristin would track the internal sensations that would arise when it felt okay to have eye contact and when it didn't feel okay. And when it didn't, she'd gently assert that boundary by asking me to avert my eyes. This gave her system a new experience of entrainment as she began to form agency over what her eyes did and did not want to see. We playfully practiced emotional mirroring, making faces at each other that the other would repeat. We would recall moments in her past in which there was a disconnection or rupture with someone, an experience that would trigger her eyes to impulsively look down and away. She'd work on slowly allowing her eyes to soften in a way that was tolerable, and then she'd look up, sometimes resting her gaze not on my eyes but on my upper right or left shoulder. This began to open the door for connection.

Over the course of many months, Kristin's ability to give and receive and connect with her eyes became profoundly stronger. Not only was there a remarkable difference in our resonance in our sessions, but her ability to connect more deeply with others saw major improvement as well.

It Takes a Village

During his attachment research, Bowlby discovered that nurturing didn't have to fall entirely on the mother's shoulders. According to his research, infants instinctually create a limited hierarchy of attachments to both ensure emotional organization and also provide backup support. Although the primary attachment figure is typically a parent, Bowlby found that children can form secure attachments with various caregivers, including older siblings, fathers, grandparents, and even non-family members like babysitters. Trauma researcher Dr. Gabor Maté says, "It takes a village of attachments to raise a child."

Healthy intimacy and human connection are pivotal in addressing many of the world's challenges, yet our culture today is marked by profound disconnection. Our modern lifestyle has divorced us from nature and traditional ways of communal living. Looking to indigenous wisdom offers insights into natural human behaviors. In hunter-gatherer societies, community was paramount, newborns were cared for by the entire tribe, and multiple lactating mothers supported the breastfeeding and nurturing journey of the child. Unlike our current nuclear family structure (and even that is falling apart), these societies embraced an extended family model embedded within an even larger supportive community.

Until recently in our history, we, too, raised our children in a supportive village—our tribe, our clan, our extended family, our community, our neighborhood. However, today in post-industrial North America, modern economic and social culture don't seem to support the importance of the relationship between children and the adults who take care of them. In previous generations, sit-down meals, family walks and games (not on computers or devices), and meaningful conversations in the home were the norm. Yet you could argue that our busy, high-tech, modern world promotes the opposite. As a result, the most important factor in child development—relationship and attachment to our caregivers—is increasingly under threat. We see this in the way that children are separated from their caregivers as both parents work overtime to earn an income that supports the high costs of living; in the way that children are being raised in single-parent homes; and in the way that children are isolated from society as they mindlessly consume what's on their phones, TV, the internet, and video games.

We look at the children of today, who are showing the highest rates of behavioral, mental, and physical illness we've ever seen—and think they need medication, more structure, or more rigid guidelines and rules. When, in reality, what they really need is strong relationships and attachment. The good news is that it's never too late to heal our attachment histories. With intention, we can reclaim this foundation for ourselves and for our children.

Childhood Attachment Styles

In the attachment theory framework, Bowlby proposed that babies are born with an internal attachment behavioral system, which is triggered in response to perceived threats. When frightened, hurt, or distressed, infants seek their primary caregiver for comfort and track through the brain and body for three things:

1. Is my caregiver *near*? Can I sense their presence? Are they physically near me? *Or . . . are my parents separated or divorced, passed on, hospitalized, incarcerated, or constantly away at work, for instance?*

2. Is my caregiver *attentive*? If they're near, do they give me attention? *Or . . . are they consumed with their own stress, mental health issues, trauma, work, or substance abuse, for instance?*

3. Is my caregiver *responsive*? When I'm in distress, do they respond in a way that is attuned and calming (like soothing and rocking me)? *Or . . . do they become angry, anxious, or disconnected from me, for instance?*

If the baby *consistently* experiences an affirmed yes to these questions, then the child will form a subconscious belief that the caregiver is reliable and safe, thereby forming a secure attachment.

Insecure Attachment

Anything other than a consistent yes to the above three questions will create an insecure attachment, which can be categorized into three predictable styles: insecure resistant (also called ambivalent or anxious), insecure avoidant, and insecure disorganized.

Insecure Resistant

If, on average, there is an *inconsistent yes*—meaning that sometimes the caregiver is near, attentive, and responsive but sometimes they're not—then the baby learns to be hypervigilant with the unpredictable attachment figure. They will seek out the caregiver and cling to them. This is because they sense that they *can* be reliable, yet they don't show up reliably. And they know the caregiver is capable of providing this secure base because they've experienced it intermittently before. So they oscillate between angry and anxious when the caregiver attempts to soothe them. They stay in distress, or "protest," with the ultimate goal to stay in contact with the caregiver as long as possible, because they don't know if this will be the last time they will experience this security.

Insecure Avoidant

If, on average, there is a *consistent no*—meaning that the caregiver is never near, attentive, and responsive—then the baby learns to be avoidant of the unreliable attachment figure, because they discern that the most effective way to regulate themselves is by not activating the caregiver. They have learned, repeatedly, that the caregiver will only dismiss their distress or add more anxiety. This lack of trust and bonding with the caregiver leads the child to become indifferent about the relationship, suppress their own needs and emotions, and form the belief they can only rely on themselves.

Insecure Disorganized

If, on average, there is a *consistent no*—meaning that the caregiver is never near, attentive, and responsive, and the baby has increased fear when the caregiver is near due to abuse, chaos, or neglect—then the baby does not form an organized response to meet their emotional needs, which often looks unpredictable and unstable. Sometimes the child becomes clingy or angry toward the caregiver and at other times avoidant, creating a push-and-pull dynamic where they occasionally want closeness but also fear it. This often stems from extreme environments in which the caregiver is frightening, frightened themselves, or completely detached. Because a child is instinctually wired for connection, they will impulsively seek out their caregiver when in distress. Yet when the caregiver is the individual creating the distress or threat, they also will instinctually pull away from the caregiver (which causes the push-and-pull dynamic). This pattern creates disorganization and extreme confusion in the child.

In relation to the nervous system, we can observe the correlation between states and styles, meaning each style can reflect the common emotions, feelings, thoughts, and behavioral patterns you often see associated with the states of your nervous system. Secure attachment is experienced in our ventral vagal response, insecure resistant attachment is experienced in our sympathetic fight-or-flight response, insecure avoidant attachment is experienced in our dorsal vagal response, and insecure disorganized attachment is experienced in both our sympathetic fight-or-flight response and our dorsal vagal response. These adaptive survival states carry on into adulthood, forming the predictable patterns of how we relate to others and how we self-regulate or co-regulate.

THE FOUR S'S

Another popular framework based on Bowlby's original attachment research is Dr. Dan Siegel's Four S's of Secure Attachment. The Four S's explain the factors that help a child maintain a feeling of being safe, seen, soothed, and, therefore, secure.

1. **Safe:** Making a commitment not to instill fear in the child, to create a "safe haven" or environment, to provide a space for emotional expression, and to repair and reconnect after conflict
2. **Seen:** Making a commitment to acknowledge and understand the child's experience, including how they feel and who they are
3. **Soothed:** Making a commitment to comfort the child in difficult times and in good times
4. And, therefore, **secure.**

Consistent Parenting, Not Perfect Parenting

Attachment theory emphasizes that parents can embrace imperfections and mistakes. Attachment parenting revolves around nurturing a relationship with your child rather than adhering to a rigid set of strategies. There's no need for perfection in parenting, because it's an unrealistic expectation. In fact, moments of disconnection or misunderstanding, known as "ruptures," are bound to occur. Yet, a "good enough" parent offers chances to mend these rifts and repair these ruptures, which fosters in the child a higher capacity to move through distressing moments.

Donald Winnicott, a renowned pediatrician and parent-infant therapist, introduced the concept of the "good enough mother" in 1953, following extensive observations of maternal behavior and its impact on infants. Through his studies, he found that manageable "failures" in caregiving can actually benefit babies and children, boosting their resilience. Additionally, Winnicott found that meeting the child's needs just 30 percent of the time is enough to create securely attached children. And later research by Dr. Edward Tronick revealed that parents and children are attuned only around 20 to 30 percent of the time.

This framework ultimately illustrates that attunement—an attempt to understand, and reliably and consistently stick it out together—is what holds the greatest weight in parenting. We see this when a baby cries and the caregiver goes through a list of potential solutions to resolve and soothe the child's distress. They may change the baby's diaper, then try a bottle, then change the baby's clothes, and then, as a last resort, go for a walk and finally the baby calms. More important than being the perfect parent is providing the child with a *sense* that "I will be with you in your distress," and "I'll keep attempting to understand and make it better."

So when parents "mess up," when they inadvertently disrupt the connection with their children—whether through raised voices, loss of composure, or mistakes—they have the chance to mend it. Embracing the concept of "rupture and repair" (breaking and restoring connection) in relationships offers significant opportunities for growth by demonstrating to children that relationships can withstand challenges and that all human emotions are valid and accepted.

How Attachment Shows Up in Adulthood

Secure attachment, preoccupied or anxious attachment (insecure resistant in children), dismissive attachment (insecure avoidant in children), and fearful-avoidant attachment (insecure disorganized in children)—these four attachment styles represent the habitual ways individuals form connections, which stem from childhood experiences and persist into adulthood relationships. As we've previously explored, these patterns are rooted in the quality of care received during early development.

Secure Attachment

This attachment style emerges from a caregiver who provided predictability, consistency, and trustworthiness. In adulthood, individuals with a secure attachment style exhibit adeptness in fostering meaningful relationships and navigating conflicts effectively. They tend to feel confident, safe, comfortable, and responsive and create appropriate boundaries. They commonly have a positive self-view and positive view of others.

Response when triggered: Not triggered easily.

Preoccupied/Anxious Attachment

This attachment style emerges from a caregiver who was inconsistent and unpredictable. This is a style of insecurity, high anxiety, and co-dependence. Those with anxious attachment tend to be emotionally volatile, fearful of rejection, deeply fearful of abandonment or being alone, clingy, appeasing, in need of reassurance, and romanticizing of others. They tend to have a negative self-view and a positive view of others, commonly believing their partner is the "better half" in the relationship. They often lack boundaries, making them vulnerable to hurt.

Response when triggered: Shutdown or fawn.

Dismissive Attachment

This attachment style emerges from a caregiver who was disengaged, distant, and unavailable. Those with dismissive attachment don't trust easily, build walls, and can be withdrawn and emotionally unresponsive. They value self-sufficiency, often pushing away those who "smother them." They tend to have a positive self-view and a negative view of others, further enforcing their hyper-independence.

Response when triggered: Flight or shutdown.

Fearful-Avoidant Attachment

This attachment style emerges from a caregiver who was chaotic and abusive, or neglectful. This is a style of total confusion surrounding relationships, where the adult oscillates between helpless and hopeless. This can be seen in heightened emotions like fear, irritability, or anger, and subdued feelings of defeat, despair, or depression. Additionally, individuals often replicate relational dynamics learned during childhood, either by selecting abusive partners or exhibiting abusive behaviors themselves. They may behave unpredictably (pushing and pulling in relationships) due to their internal biological conflict between a desire for intimacy and fear of it. They tend to have a negative self-view and a negative view of others.

Response when triggered: Varies (fight, flight, shutdown, fawn).

Earned Secure Attachment

We experience attachment on a continuum, and we develop a combination of different strategies. In other words, you are not just one style, you are *all* styles. Just as your nervous system has a dominant protective state (do you tend to fight, flee, or shut down?), so, too, does your attachment.

This is why you might notice that you have a mixture of secure and insecure styles. The question is, which style is behind the wheel *most of the time*? If you find that an insecure style (either anxious, dismissive, or fearful-avoidant) runs the show, you're not alone. In fact, more than 50 percent of the population has a dominant insecure attachment style.

The aim of attachment healing isn't to extinguish these responses, but to become more securely attached so that your dominant state is not under the insecure attachment umbrella. Today, my style is roughly around 80 percent secure, 10 percent anxious, 5 percent dismissive, and 5 percent fearful-avoidant. Yet this wasn't always the case—my secure attachment was "earned."

The good news is, although our attachment style follows a predictable path, with time and intentional effort to change, attachment is relatively fluid. It's not set in stone, just set in place. This is the framework behind *earned secure attachment*, when a person develops a secure attachment style in adulthood after overcoming attachment insecurity from childhood.

The other piece of good news is that you can heal your attachment history within *new attachments* or relationships you find yourself in today. This means you don't have to trek the painful path back to childhood or mend your attachment wounds alongside caregivers who cannot or will not do so. Ultimately, the interpersonal connections you create today have the power to foster new attachments or repair old ones.

Secure attachment can be cultivated through a deep and enduring bond with a surrogate attachment figure who helps build a new relational foundation and secure base. This transformative attachment can arise within or outside a romantic relationship, meaning you can earn security through a partner, friend, mentor, or even therapist. The process can take time—research shows that it will take up to three to five years of experiencing a newly secure relationship for similar positive expectations of other relationships to form. Yet studies also demonstrate that it takes just one secure relationship to change your attachment style. This earned secure attachment hinges on relationships with the self and others. For instance, earning a secure attachment with yourself depends on the repairing of your relationship with yourself, whereas earning secure attachment with others depends on the repair with others.

From Anxious to Secure

My history of attachment wounds runs deep, even farther back than my lifetime. (I'll share more about these intergenerational attachment patterns in the next chapter.) Yet what I experienced in my earliest years also left lasting imprints that deeply and destructively impacted my relationship with myself and with others. Not only had I been exposed to trauma while in the womb—developing in a toxic soup of my mother's survival hormones and drugs—I also was taken from my mother immediately at birth, separated from her during my first few months of life, and placed in foster care. This meant there was no mother-to-infant bonding, no nursing, and no being held or soothed by her. And after we were reunited, I would spend much of my formative years emotionally and physically separated from her as she poured herself into her career.

From the outside, my childhood looked relatively normal, even to me. It wasn't until my late teens and early twenties that I recognized that my insecurities, toxic codependent patterns, and deep fear of rejection and abandonment weren't at all normal. As I began studying more about the nervous system and trauma, I was introduced to science that revealed to me my harsh reality—my own inability to care for or love myself as an adult was a direct reflection of how I was cared for as a child. I had been born into a world of hurt, with a biological father who was absent and a struggling young mother, a single parent, who had limited capacity and tools to provide the emotional and physical security I needed as an infant. As I grew older, I could sense that there were parts of my mother that felt burdened by her children. I could feel this in her repeated remarks that *if she could go back and do it over, she wouldn't have had kids when she did,* or that *she never got to experience freedom and a life for just herself,* or admitting that *motherhood was never her top priority, her career was.* And although now, as an adult, I can understand her perspective, as a young child, that was hard to hear. Later, I would discover that her mother carried similar sentiments—my mother and aunt shared that they often felt like my grandmother "didn't want to be a mother" and perhaps even "resented it."

It's been both comforting and challenging to become a parent myself. Having my children made me much more sympathetic to my mom; she was extremely young when she had my brother and me, and the cards were overwhelmingly stacked against her. I, on the other hand, didn't have my babies until I was thirty, by which point I had grown and healed a lot as an individual. I would hold my very own tiny and vulnerable babies in my arms, knowing what they needed, while also knowing that my mother couldn't give me what I needed. I've come to terms with my past—and my mother's past, because it explains so much about who she is—while also not excusing the hurt I experienced.

That's the beauty of duality in healing: a part of me was once upset and grieving, and another part of me can hold so much compassion for everything she went through. One part of me doesn't invalidate the other. They all have space to coexist.

Although my mother and I turned a reparative corner in our relationship as I came into adulthood, the gift in attachment healing means that my attachment wounds as a child could be tended to and mended in any secure relationship, not just with her. Relational wounds require relational healing. I needed to give my nervous system different experiences of connection—experiences that felt safe, comforting, and consistent. In this case, that healing happened through my relationship with my husband, David. Yet it wasn't an easy road at the beginning. They say opposites tend to attract, and the same can be said when it comes to attachment styles: David has a default dismissive style, while I have a default anxious style; he came into the relationship hyper-independent, and I came in with codependent tendencies. This dynamic is common, because we often seek out the types of partners who trigger our dominant and familiar state. In this case, David had subconsciously sought out a partner who would "smother" him, pushing him farther into exile in the relationship. Whereas I subconsciously sought out a partner who would feel "distant and detached," further heightening my fear of abandonment and impulse to cling tighter. And although we loved each other deeply, the early chapters of our relationship were anything but harmonious.

At the time, I had become chronically codependent of others, jumping from one serious relationship to the next, terrified of being alone. Relationships would consume me because a deep fear of abandonment guided my anxious and insecure tendencies. It should come as no surprise then that I attracted people who kept me there, whether it was someone who was emotionally abusive, someone who was emotionally unavailable, someone who needed fixing or saving or who needed me to take care of them (creating a dynamic where they'd never leave), or someone who seemed distant and disinterested (triggering my impulse to cling and chase). Naturally, because David was more of an avoidant and independent person, when we first started dating, that's what initially attracted me to him. It didn't take long to understand why he had closed off parts of himself to the rest of the world. He grew up an only child, with a father who was emotionally and physically distant and who left him and his mother when David was thirteen after she had given him an ultimatum—*us or the alcohol*.

Although our opposite styles often clashed, over time we each provided the other with experiences that softened our insecure styles, eventually meeting each other in the middle where earned secure attachment would be born. I showed him slowly over time that he could be vulnerable, he could be interdependent, and that he would be met with attunement and loyalty. And he showed me slowly over time that I could trust him to stay through the good and the bad and that I was worthy of love. I remember contemplating whether I wanted to accept a position to work overseas, meaning that I would be separated from him for nearly six months. I was terrified to leave, but the commitment and reassurance he had given during our first three years together was enough to allow myself some independence. I remember his exact words when I came to him with my hesitation about leaving: "You know I'll be here when you get back. You owe it to yourself to live a life outside of this relationship. Because at the end of the day, I can complement your life but I can't complete you—only you can do that. You need to learn to love yourself more than you love me." Had it not been for the tending and nurturing of our relationship that had preceded that moment, I don't know that I ever would have taken the leaps I did in my career. His steady behavior taught my nervous system that it was safe to experience something new, and to expect that same safety and attunement moving forward. His warm and consistent love set the new standard.

REPARENTING YOUR YOUNGER SELF

Becoming a parent granted me an incredible opportunity to continue to heal my previous attachment wounds. Your brain remains fluid and capable of developing new connections every day of your life. It's the most pliable in childhood; 90 percent of your brain is developed by the time you're age three or four. The second season of life that provides the most plasticity in your brain is when you become a parent for the first time, because your brain is being triggered and mirrored by your baby's experiences. It's as if you get to experience your childhood all over again. You're able to learn, play, and connect in ways you perhaps couldn't back then. This kind of healing has been one of the most profound aspects of my parenting journey. I've been able to witness and experience childlike wonder through the eyes of my little ones, while also leaning into the love, affection, and warmth that I often longed for in my own childhood. That little Brittany is still within me, and she gets to experience this chapter of life alongside my children and adult Brittany. Peter Levine was right: it's truly never too late to give yourself the childhood you deserve.

The Wound, from a Somatic Lens

Attachment trauma in childhood can lead to deep-rooted beliefs in adulthood of being damaged, unlovable, or unable to trust others (even yourself). Feelings of shame, unworthiness, and helplessness may partner with these beliefs, along with anxiety and a sense of not belonging. Eventually, these feelings of insecurity and inadequacy can shape your identity, your relationships, and your capacity to live within your own body.

An attachment wound or injury is considered both a developmental trauma and a relational trauma. In other words, this relational trauma (a rupture) happens in the developmental stage and, therefore, affects how the child is able to process the trauma, often arresting development (emotional, psychological, cognitive, and physical). The goal in healing attachment trauma through a somatic lens is to focus on *regulation* and *repair,* where we aim to develop nervous system and emotional regulation and also focus on relational rupture and repair cycles. By doing so, we create a better internal relationship with our emotions and lean into new opportunities for connection with ourselves and others. Note that in the commitment to making this work, gentle and titrated steps for healing attachment wounds will be explored more deeply in part II of this book. For now, here is a basic overview.

The intention behind *regulation* is to build the autonomic nervous system and emotional self. Attachment is an *emotional* experience (emotional bond), so the quality of our attachment in childhood has a direct correlation to the state of our internal emotional world today. Our emotions may be extreme and unbearable (what we refer to as "Global High Intensity Activation"), or they may be absent, dissociated, or disowned. For example, if we experienced repeated misattunement, neglect, or abuse in childhood, then we'll likely hold grief, disappointment, rage, and shame in our body and physiology—potentially creating denial about love or resistance to having our own wants or needs. In addition, if there was abuse during childhood by a loved one, our involuntary survival impulses to run away or fight back were likely overridden, because those responses could have created further harm or hurt. This can create an internal landscape where our thwarted fight response of anger or our thwarted flight response of fear may become either intensely experienced and projected in the present day or inaccessible and dissociated.

After first bringing our awareness and access to our supportive resources of the present, we then gently improve our ability to be with our emotional experience in the here and now, first just by noticing, not by expressing. This means the initial step is building the capacity to sense and identify our feelings. As we begin to learn this language of our body and physiology, we can start to bring special attention to accurate reflections and expressions of our emotions so they can finally be met with attunement (understanding and compassion), either from ourselves or others. This is where the *repair* from previous ruptures can begin to take place.

Here, through self-attunement and attunement with others, we can rebuild our patterns of connection, grow our faith in ourselves and others, and begin to restore a sense of personal power and agency—helping us improve our boundaries and advocate for our wants and needs.

You'll learn in part II how to use Somatic Experiencing to connect you to the felt sense of emotion—the interoceptive underpinnings (sensations) of emotion—which helps release the survival charge held within those intense emotions (like the anger and fear mentioned above) and tap into practices that help you build capacity and resilience in your nervous system. You'll also learn how to access healthy aggression—your innate life force (fight response) that may have been crippled in your formative years—allowing you to rise into your power.

Reflection: Self-Attunement for Beginners

Self-attunement involves the capacity to understand and respond to our own internal emotional states, needs, and perspectives. It marks the initial step toward reshaping our perception of self as we grow. This skill can be nurtured through mindfulness, self-compassion techniques, and therapeutic interventions, such as the Internal Family Systems (IFS) model, created by Richard C. Schwartz. Using IFS, we can utilize the tools of *parts work* to attune to the parts of us that carry our attachment history. Unresolved attachment trauma often resides within the younger, wounded parts of the self, commonly known as the inner child. These are the irrational and hurt parts that come to the surface when we're triggered or in pain. You may at times feel closely connected to these vulnerable parts of you, while at other times you may feel more connected to your regulated adult self, who provides a sense of strength and confidence.

In the spirit of self-attunement, you can allow these younger parts to feel understood, soothed, and supported by your more regulated and resilient adult self. For instance, as an adult, you now can make choices that were unavailable to you during your childhood: the option to express how you feel, to set boundaries, and to walk away, to name a few. Your adult self can foster experiences that your younger self never received—like moments of compassion, curiosity, clarity, creativity, calm, confidence, courage, and connectedness (based on the eight C's of IFS)—showing these younger parts that you openheartedly want to get to know them. You also have the understanding that when these painful feelings present themselves, you can be reminded that these are imprints of painful experiences that are now over and in the past. With this awareness, you can compassionately attune the needs and emotions of your inner child.

Here are some prompts for self-attunement:

1. Envision yourself as a child. It might even help to look at an actual photo of younger you. Can you imagine what it would be

like to sit across from that younger you now, to be in connection while taking a few deep breaths together?

2. If you struggle to feel warmth or kindness toward your younger self, can you instead visualize someone who could serve as a safe ally for this inner child, either someone you know, a fictitious character, or someone you admire or look up to? Picture this person offering a loving or compassionate gaze to that vulnerable part of you.

3. Now, can you imagine your adult self or safe ally befriending or speaking kindly to your younger self? Do they offer words of comfort, unconditional acceptance, protection, or reassurance to your inner child?

Note that if you encounter difficulties during this practice, you can always come back to this reflection at any time.

Reflection: Cues of Connection

For those who have attachment wounds, it's sometimes easier to recount our caregivers' shortcomings or negative attributes than remember moments of connection. As creatures of survival, that's only natural. We're good at recognizing feelings of hurt so we can protect ourselves from that same hurt in the future. However, it's equally as important to develop a radar for cues of connection. This helps us highlight what supports and benefits us in our lives.

Why is this important? Because your nervous system *prioritizes* connection and social engagement as a means to regulate. Remember that our ventral state is one of safety and connection. The better our capacity to be in connection with others, the more regulated our nervous system becomes. This doesn't mean ignoring our traumas and wounds from the past—we can honor the duality of *both* wounds and connection. By bringing to life supportive imagery and memories, we can orient the resources that supported us then into the now. Connecting with experiences of co-regulation long enough allows us to alter old neural pathways, get unstuck from states of survival, and enhance our ability to access secure attachment.

With this in mind, what are the times in your life that you felt supported, cared for, or attuned to? What did that care look like? Who provided it for you—a caregiver, sibling, extended family, friend, teacher, coworker, etc.? As you consider this moment, can you notice your internal experience? Are there glimmers of emotion, sensation, or impulse that speak to this supportive memory?

Practice: Boundary and Touch Work

When attachment wounds are deep, our ability to be comforted through touch, by ourselves or by others, can become damaged. This guided practice gently explores your relationship to touch.

First, start by closing your eyes, if it feels comfortable. Begin to imagine a recent moment that was *mildly* difficult, perhaps running late to a meeting, having a disagreement with someone, etc. As you recall this moment, is there a place in your body that is calling to you for self-touch or comfort? This could be placing a hand on your heart, clasping your hands together, hugging your arms, rubbing your legs, and more. Can you place a hand there? As your hand settles, can you begin to notice how that is for you? Does it provide support in the body or further discomfort? If discomfort arises, what would it be like to pull away your hand?

Now, how would it be to imagine someone in your life, who you feel safe and connected to, joining your hand with theirs? Can you track within your body what happens? Is there a sigh of relief? Is there more overwhelm? If there's overwhelm, what would it be like to imagine them pulling away their hand?

If their hand felt supportive, how would it be now to imagine that they give supportive touch to that place on your body with their own hand, such as a hand on your shoulder, giving you a hug, or holding your hand? Have space to feel your body's answer, knowing that there is no right or wrong response.

Now, how would it be to imagine them pulling away their hand? Does it feel too fast, too slow, or too abrupt? How does your body show you that? Recognize that how we leave a moment of connection or a relational experience is just as important as how we enter.

How would it be now to imagine touching that safe person, such as walking up to them with open and inviting arms, leaning your head on their shoulder, or reaching for their hand?

Throughout this exercise, were there patterns from your body that whispered where there was a no and where there was a yes? This could have been felt as a constriction in the muscles, a held breath, heat, or a racing heart. It could have been ease and relaxation in the body, deeper access to breathing, or settling of the heart. Can you say, "Thank you, body, for letting me know how you do and don't want to be touched. That makes sense, given what you've lived through"?

ATTACHMENT QUIZ

Curious about what your attachment style is? Feel free to take the free attachment quiz from attachment expert and therapist Dr. Diane Poole Heller by visiting traumasolutions.com/attachment-styles-quiz.

CHAPTER 7

The Armor of Trauma and the Five Stuck Personalities

Every human has a true authentic self. Trauma is the disconnection from it and healing is the reconnection to it.
—Dr. Gabor Maté

You've seen the term *armor* nearly twenty times in this book, because I often use the phrase "armored up" to describe how your well-intentioned nervous system goes into states of protection. To really illustrate this, let's imagine this physiological shield to be a full knight's suit of armor. Whenever you're in a traumatic situation, as you know, your nervous system is going to have an automatic response. It senses danger, so to protect you, it says, in essence, *We're going to armor up and go into battle so you can survive.* If, after the battle, there's an absence of a felt sense of safety in your body or environment (including from those around you), then you won't be able to take off the armor—in other words, you won't be able to complete the threat response cycle. An example of this could be having your painful experiences dismissed, ignored, or invalidated.

For many of us, we either inherited our armor from generations before us or acquired it in our earliest years of life, before we could even remember a time without it, making this armor all we've ever known. For others, a traumatic experience can bring about this new suit of armor. And when stuck in perpetual states of survival, we can lose ourselves in its defensive walls, as if losing contact—if we even had it to begin with—to the authentic person underneath. It's on this battlefield that we become unrecognizable to others, and even to ourselves, as we take on personalities that don't feel natural to who we are. Over time, this armor that was once meant to help us survive the trauma eventually becomes more like a burden, as our now not-so-shining-armor seems to create more self-destruction in our lives than self-protection.

What can feel even more defeating is when your armor comes cloaked as a diagnosis or disorder, rather than being seen and treated as a very *natural response* to help you survive an unnatural or overwhelming experience. For instance, instead of post-traumatic stress *disorder*, obsessive-compulsive *disorder* (OCD), or bipolar *disorder*, we could reason these to be a post-traumatic stress *response*, an obsessive-compulsive *response*, or a bipolar *response*. These "disorders," among the numerous others that we see in the *Diagnostic and Statistical Manual of Mental Disorders* (DSM), were more often than not the adaptations and coping mechanisms intricately and brilliantly created by your brain and biology to help you manage what once overcame your capacity. This isn't to invalidate these very real and often very debilitating disorders. Yet recognizing that they are the armor and natural response to trauma can give us more agency and power in our abilities to self-heal.

Somatic Experiencing allows us to slowly and gently remove the protective physiological armor of the past, granting us the ability to rediscover who we are before the trauma told us who to be. We do this by first catching up and reconnecting to the safety of the present, followed by building our capacity to be with our bodies through both expansion (what feels good) and contraction (what doesn't feel good), and then finally allowing the nervous system to process and complete in the here and now what was too overwhelming to process back then. This is how we gently remove the armor and return to the ventral state of safety and connection at the top of the ladder.

It's important to remember that in true somatic fashion, we must shed these layers in a way that's *titrated*. For instance, when considering your full suit of armor, you don't take off the armor all at once. Remember that your nervous system operates from the belief that "same equals safe." Therefore, it will always prioritize what's familiar, and it will always resist change, even if it's "good for us." (Reminder: Your nervous system doesn't operate from the rational/thinking brain!) So if that armor is what's familiar, then stripping it all at once will be met with further activation and overwhelm. To prevent that from happening, you'll slowly remove one piece at a time, allowing the parts of you below to feel safer with each plate removed. You'll hold compassion and maybe even gratitude for your armor while also recognizing you're no longer fighting that battle anymore.

The Five Stuck Personalities

As you just read, our armor can hinder us more than help us when we have unprocessed trauma from the past. The prolonged charge of stress hormones and an incomplete nervous system response can keep us stuck in a vicious loop of survival as these maladaptive coping behaviors become our normal. These are the subconscious procedural patterns and implicit memories of the body being played out in the here and now—the way we minimize, run away, catastrophize, blow up, and avoid. Over time, these deeply wired impulsive patterns that rule our lives begin to feel as if they're a certain type of *personality* we've grown into.

Copious research has been done through the years comparing personality and individuality. Individuality is who we are at our core. Personality, which is created in our earliest years of life, is the person we had to become, or the masks or armor we had to wear, so we could survive by fitting in with our tribe. This includes, perhaps, how we learned as infants to shut down or suppress our emotions because they were often met with dysregulation from our caregivers, creating disconnection to our lifeline, our attachment figure (the person with whom we carry our deepest emotional bond). As Dr. Gabor Maté explains, "People have two needs: attachment and authenticity. When authenticity threatens attachment, attachment trumps authenticity."[1] In other words, in our earliest years—when connection to our authentic self threatens connection to our attachment figure—we will almost always sacrifice connection to self.

The personality versus individuality research also mirrors the age-old debate of nature versus nurture—our authentic and true self is our nature, and our prevailing conditioned self is our nurture. When stuck in our armor, we become caught between the two—nature versus nurture, personality versus individuality. We grapple with "life before trauma" and "life after trauma." Even more, for those of us who perhaps never had a "life before trauma," we confront our armor with *Who was I meant to be, without you here?*

What's important to know is that our armor serves a purpose and, therefore, isn't to be discarded. Instead, perhaps envision that you're able to melt your armor and forge a smaller shield that can come to your aid when similar threats present themselves. In other words, if you're stuck wearing an armor that represents your *fight* response— although the goal is to express and expel whatever previous fight response wasn't allowed to be completed in the past—you don't want to completely do away with the fight response moving forward because it's a necessity in managing everyday challenges and activation. Altogether, each nervous system state holds vital responses that support us in our day-to-day lives—it's not bad to set a boundary with someone who wrongs you (fight), or to need to work long hours when a project deadline is coming up (flight), or to crave some alone time bingeing our favorite TV series for a day (shutdown), or to go out of our way to help others (fawn). The goal isn't to eradicate these parts of us, but to metaphorically place them in the backseat so our regulated self can finally take the reins. We want our armor to support us, not suffocate us. Sometimes our really smart survival strategies just need some major updating.

One of the primary goals of Somatic Experiencing is to help people complete incomplete trauma responses or experiences, to get them out of these stuck states. It's important to explain that although each nervous system state will look, sound, and feel *unique* to each person (you will be identifying yours in your Polyvagal Personal Profile Map soon), here are some commonalities we often see with each of the five stuck personalities.

1. Fight

This is the state of anger, aggression, and control.

Behavior Characteristics

These often are people who are viewed as either explosive, resentful, irritable, narcissistic, or bullying, with a dose of self-entitlement and self-preservation. They can be controlling, demeaning, combative, manipulative, demanding, defensive, dismissive or criticizing of others, quick to anger, and hot-tempered.

What You'll Hear

"I'm right, you're wrong, and here's why . . ."

"I just like to be in control."

"That's not fair!"

"If I'm angry it's because you made me."

How It Shows Up in Relationships

A communication style that often presents as talking over the other person, inability to listen, gaslighting or manipulative, deflective, reactive, controlling of others, and aggressive. Rarely takes accountability or apologizes. Leaves the other person feeling like they have to walk on eggshells and are never heard.

How You Carry It in Your Body
The hallmarks of a sympathetic fight response are hypervigilance; a puffed-up posture; the impulse to move toward, defend, or attack; a rigid spine; and bracing and tension within the muscles due to the presence of the increased stress hormones adrenaline and cortisol. Other characteristics include heightened scanning of the environment through sight (dilated pupils) and sound (activated low ear muscles) to defend from potential threat. Emotional expression amplified (tears or vocalized expression). Increased heart rate, respiration, blood pressure, and stimulation of sweat glands. Relaxation of the bladder. Inhibition or slowing down of the reproductive system, immune system, digestive system, and insulin activity. Nausea or butterflies as blood motility is directed away from the stomach and to your muscles and limbs for action-taking. Lightheaded or dizzy as a result of faster breathing.

Disorder or Response?
Common diagnosis (or misdiagnosis): narcissistic personality disorder, oppositional defiant disorder, conduct disorder, or intermittent explosive disorder.

When I Was in the Fight State
This was me after my assault. In the two years between the incident and the trial, I was drinking a lot to cope. I had morphed from being a sweet-natured and gentle person to someone with an abundance of bitterness and anger to go around—anger that I had zero clue what to do with, until the intoxication would take over and it would attempt to get released in aggressive outbursts. Looking back now, I can validate that although it could have been expressed in much healthier ways, that anger was righteous and valid for a number of reasons.

As I've shared, I had been physically overpowered during the assault when I attempted to fight back, which created an incomplete fight response within my nervous system, leaving behind a toxic and poisonous environment of adrenaline-fueled rage that showed up in my everyday life. In addition, the victim-blaming from those closest to me left a lasting impression of distrust of others and the need to armor up, even against the people I loved most. Lastly, the judicial process had become interminably painful for a number of reasons, including the fact that over the course of those two years, my trial was postponed (or "continued") nine times.

A trial's continuance often happens in cases where the evidence is overwhelming—the defense will strategically drag out the trial process to break down the victim with the hopes that they'll settle for a plea deal or drop the charges entirely. This meant that nine times, during a two-year period, I had to meet with my attorneys to "rehearse" for trial. Each time, I had to go through my taped statements and depositions before practice being on the witness stand. Nine times I had to relive every graphic detail of that night. Nine times I strapped on that armor for a dress rehearsal to finally take back my power . . . only to get a call the day before trial to learn that I'd yet again prepared for a battle that wasn't going to come to an end anytime soon. It was re-traumatizing, to say the least. But I kept telling myself that after my perpetrator was behind bars I would feel better.

However, that wasn't the case. And as you've already learned, it was that fight response that placed me in a jail cell less than thirty days after the sentencing.

2. Flight
This is the state of fear, anxiety, panic, and hypervigilance.

Behavior Characteristics
Here, you overcompensate for most things in an attempt to resolve the overwhelm of mobilizing hormones that help you flee. You overachieve, overanalyze, and overperform. It's where you *go go go* because you need

to *do do do* to stay distracted. You practice escapism through busyness either with work, your newest hobbies, or obsessions; excessive use of substances; or compulsive behaviors that provide temporary relief, like gambling, shopping, or even sex. You're subconsciously attracted to stress and hold the highest standards of perfectionism for yourself. You're running away and avoiding people, places, and situations that create any discomfort. You're restless and, therefore, find it difficult to be present, pay attention, or slow down.

What You'll Hear

"I don't want to deal with this."

"Let's talk about something else."

"I just want to get out of here."

"I'm just a type A personality."

How It Shows Up in Relationships

A communication style that often presents as avoiding relationships, deflecting or running away from hard conversations, cutting people off or stonewalling, unable to handle conflict, struggling with commitment, and feelings of being trapped.

How You Carry It in Your Body

The hallmarks of a sympathetic flight response are turning away, the impulse to escape or move away, a rigid spine, and bracing and tension within the muscles due to the presence of the increased stress hormones adrenaline and cortisol. Other characteristics include heightened scanning of the environment through sight (dilated pupils) and sound (activated low ear muscles) to flee from potential threat. Emotional expression amplified (tears or vocalized expression). Increased heart rate, respiration, blood pressure, and stimulation of sweat glands. Relaxation of the bladder. Inhibition or slowing down of the reproductive system, immune system, digestive system, and insulin activity. Nausea or butterflies as blood motility is directed away from the stomach and to your muscles and limbs for action-taking. Light-headed or dizzy as a result of faster breathing.

Disorder or Response?

Common diagnosis (or misdiagnosis): anxiety disorder, obsessive-compulsive personality disorder, bipolar disorder, attention deficit hyperactivity disorder, or panic disorder.

When I Was in the Flight State

During my roughest years of recovery, and in the rarer moments when I'm not anchored in ventral, my home-away-from-home state is flight. It's where I run away from life by filling my schedule; becoming engrossed and distracted with my newest obsessions, projects, or ideas; and feeling the need to be an overachieving perfectionist. It's also where I used to lean on substances to escape. The root of this dominant response can be easily traced back through the generational line of women in my maternal family—and the apparent abandonment wound we all seemingly inherited.

From my great-great grandmother on, we've all hoisted the armor of flight. And with that armor came a set of specific subconscious limiting beliefs, with the most important being that to survive, "We had to learn to stand alone," as my grandmother states. This meant placing extreme value on our independence as women because each of us would come to believe that we could only depend on ourselves, as others would eventually leave us or let us down. Based on the circumstances, this personality made a lot of sense.

Not only had my great-great-grandmother been a young widow, but my great-grandmother also lost her husband in the Battle of the Bulge in 1944. My grandmother had just turned four years old. Although my great-grandmother remarried shortly after her husband's passing to a man who would abuse her, she had already begun the process of figuring out life on her own. She began working multiple jobs—in a time when women were expected to be home with the children—and eventually became a wildly successful real estate investor. Taking her independence into her own hands, she became a "go-getter" to those around her. But in the home, she would retreat from her children and became a habitual smoker, which would ultimately become so detrimental to her health that it led to her death.

My grandmother didn't just inherit that armor, but she also had it reaffirmed by her own experiences of abandonment and disappointment. This included the loss of her father, followed subsequently by her stepfather's abuse, and then becoming trapped in her own marriage that was laden with deceit and decades of infidelity. In pursuit of survival, she, too, broke the mold of the "average woman" for her time. She received her law degree (graduating magna cum laude at the top of her class), established her own financial wealth via a lucrative investment career in real estate, and even became an outspoken advocate for women's rights while joining the pioneering feminist movement in the times of Gloria Steinem. Yet behind the facade, she also faced an inner turmoil that pushed her headfirst into self-medicating, depression, and suicidal ideation—making herself often inaccessible and detached as a mother, holed up in her bedroom throughout the day and then drinking throughout the night. Recognizing she was "trapped" in her marriage, she started seeking answers and the meaning of life outside it.

It's no surprise my mother had a similar trajectory. Designated as "gifted," from an early age she was put into advanced classes and enrolled in accelerated educational programs. She grew up excelling in sports and ultimately learned that achievement and high performance would bring her the praise and attention she didn't otherwise receive from an often-absent mother and a father who was too busy being a captain in the Navy and running a legal practice. By early high school, she was one of the best softball pitchers in the state of California. She was the "golden child" of her two siblings. Then, she met my father.

At seventeen, she became pregnant with my brother, dropped out of high school, and moved in with her boyfriend. It was two years later, when she was pregnant with me, that she discovered that my father had been seeing another woman, a woman he then left my mother for. Now pregnant and a single mom with nowhere to go, she and my brother would either stay with friends or sleep in her car while living off food stamps. It was the ultimate betrayal. She had sacrificed everything for this man, only to be abandoned. She was a young mother (really still just a child herself), alone, with pain that became too much to bear. Pain that she was never given the tools to process. By putting on the familiar armor passed down by her mother, she ultimately succumbed to substances to escape her dark reality. And we already know what would follow—my birth, when I was forcibly taken from her and placed into foster care because methamphetamine was found in my system.

It didn't take my mother long after my birth to right her wrongs and get her life back on track. What was already laid out before her and hardwired into her heritage was the determination to never depend on anyone again. She worked incredibly hard, excelling in her profession and breaking gender barriers. Yet eventually she made her work her life and everything else—her kids, her marriage, and her health included—secondary. Work became her escape when life became too much. It didn't leave her, it kept her distracted, and it gave her worth. It even brought her comfort immediately after my brother died, allowing her to quickly bury her grief. And work wasn't the only thing that kept her detached from her feelings and running away from the pain of the past. The numbing had transformed over the years from drugs, to food, to alcohol. This armor became so destructive that she'd have to have multiple health procedures to repair the damage of these addictions. When she was diagnosed with cancer, that was finally the wake-up call that would transform her life. Realizing her thick-plated armor was now poisoning her, for the first time in her life she began to peel back the layers of unresolved and unprocessed pain from the past. It was then that she began to heal in remarkable ways.

As my aunt (my mother's sister) so poignantly shared with me, "We [the women in our family] can put on a good front, but sometimes we're just little girls who want love and approval." It's this fear of being abandoned, rejected, or disappointed that created this mask of flight response in us all.

3. Shutdown

This is the state of overwhelm, shame, and hopelessness.

Behavior Characteristics

This is the "emergency brake" of the nervous system when circumstances become too overwhelming. Shutdown commonly looks like exhaustion, isolation, lack of emotion, depression, lack of self-care or motivation, "laziness," dissociation, numbness, brain fog and confusion, lack of memory, procrastination, bingeing (TV, internet, food, or substances), and increased sleeping patterns. People often end up in shutdown due to two reasons. One is life circumstances—an experience or upbringing where perhaps there was abuse, neglect, or lack of emotional regulation from the caretaker that created an armor of suppression and disconnection. Second is being in a fight-or-flight state for too long, causing the nervous system to "burn out" and shut down to conserve energy.

What You'll Hear

"I don't care."

"Uh . . ." (Little to no response or engagement.)

"Life will always be this way."

"I deserve this."

How It Shows Up in Relationships

A communication style that often presents as little to no expression of emotion, spacing out or having a hard time being present in conversations, lack of acknowledgment or response, acting like they don't care, the feeling of being distant, and decreased physical touch and eye contact.

How You Carry It in Your Body

The hallmarks of a parasympathetic shutdown response are a collapsed and slouched spine to hide you or make you small, along with loose muscles. Other characteristics include decreased scanning and awareness of threat, instead presenting as a downward gaze or blank stare. Sensory information goes offline (halting at the thalamus) as endorphins release to numb pain and dynorphins release, allowing you to dissociate from your inner and external world. Decreased heart rate, respiration, blood pressure, and body temperature. Pale and cold skin and limbs as blood motility moves to the core to keep the vital organs supported for "hibernation." Little to no movement as the body enters a state of immobilization and conservation, while insulin activity and fuel storage increase. Inhibition or slowing down of the reproductive system and immune system.

Disorder or Response?

Common diagnosis (or misdiagnosis): major depressive disorder, attention deficit disorder, dissociative identity disorder, or schizophrenia.

When I Was in the Shutdown State

In the hustle of the modern world, we often find ourselves succumbing to the pressure to do everything and be everything—and this is especially true for women. This pressure is something I've explored deeply through the reflection of the "solo separate self" and our cultural glorification of fierce independence. This belief, as I shared earlier, was passed down through generations of women in my family and deeply influenced my life and views.

However, the truth I've come to realize—and something I'm passionate about sharing—is that the notion of being a superwoman is not only unrealistic but also damaging. Women are often told we can have it all—career success, a wonderful relationship or marriage, a perfect family life, financial independence, and more. But in reality, when we push too hard in one area, other aspects of our life invariably suffer. This message sticks out in the 2014 commencement speech at Dartmouth, when Shonda Rhimes (creator of *Grey's Anatomy* and other successful TV shows) shared about the myth of *women having it all*. She stated, "People ask me, Shonda, how do you do it all? The answer is this: I don't. Whenever you see me succeeding in one area of my life, that almost certainly means I am failing in another area of my life."[2]

For me, this realization hit hard during a period in my professional life when I became incredibly burnt out. At the time I was a brand-new mother, juggling multiple careers and the financial pressure to provide for my family after my husband lost his job due to the pandemic. The more my businesses grew, the more life felt increasingly overwhelming.

I saw how my career demands impacted the time and energy I could devote to myself, my marriage, and my children. I was spent, with nothing left to give. Stuck in shutdown and burnout, I went into a season of withdrawal from myself and from others. I struggled with insomnia and fatigue, disabling me from leaning into the life-affirming activities that had always helped me feel better, like exercise and co-regulation. It didn't take long for me to become a mere shell of myself, finding it hard to just get through the workday.

This was a turning point in my career, leading me to reshape my businesses to better support the life I wanted—a life where I could be present and engaged with myself and my family without feeling overwhelmed by my professional responsibilities.

Self-preservation became paramount, and it also became the theme of that following year within my business. My employees and team knew this was priority number one. So I set strict work hours for all of us (no more 24/7 availability), created better boundaries, cut back on my client list, decided against posting to social media on the weekends, started conceptualizing a new format of my healing program that would give us better work-life balance, began outsourcing more of my work (like hiring an executive assistant and chief financial officer), and even set a task in our weekly team meeting for everyone on the call to share one thing they had done that week in honor of self-preservation. Over the years since, I've continued to make changes. This journey has involved hard choices, sacrifices, and letting go of certain expectations and pressures I've always placed on myself. Yet today, I'm finally at a place where I look forward to having a three-day work week so I can truly pour into myself and my family in the ways I've always dreamed.

So if you find yourself inspired by how some people manage to "do it all," know that it's a work in progress, and they don't always get it right. Yet, it is possible to create a life that truly feels worth waking up to—one that isn't overwhelming, exhausting, or dictated by others' expectations but is instead authentically yours.

4. Fawn

Fawn is the state of seeking safety through appeasing the person we sense is a perceived threat. It's a blended state of both our sympathetic flight response and our dorsal shutdown response, whereby we are mobilized by fear (flight) while also shutting down and disconnecting from our own needs, desires, and self (dorsal).

Behavior Characteristics

Here, we are guided by fear as we befriend and tend to others to avoid danger. This presents as conflict avoidance through extreme submissiveness, compliance, or being overly accommodating of others. We do this by people-pleasing, overexplaining, overapologizing, or trying to be perfect. This is where codependent tendencies can occur, where you become a chronic caregiver, savior, and/or fixer, thereby losing your identity in others you place as more important than yourself. This is also where you abandon your boundaries, avoid confrontation for the sake of keeping the peace, and say yes to anything with the hopes of being accepted—making you more prone to exploitation. When a disagreement does occur, you often retract your opinion out of fear of the consequences. You consistently defer to others to make decisions for you. You're hypersensitive to others' somatic cues and are always monitoring their emotional state for signs of threat.

What You'll Hear

"I just want everyone to be happy."

"It was my fault, I'm sorry." (Even when not at fault.)

"It's just so hard for me to say no."

"No one will like me if I don't do what they want."

How It Shows Up in Relationships

A communication style that often presents as overly kind, agreeable, and submissive. You go with the flow, because it's difficult to know or express your own needs. Lack of boundaries and apologizing when you're not at fault. Desperate to appease the other. Feeling like you're unworthy of love or flawed and will be "found out" in the relationship. There is often an extreme fear of abandonment, rejection, or ruffling feathers.

How You Carry It in Your Body

The hallmarks of a blended fawn response are disconnection from your body and possible dissociation. This dominant flight response, blended with a nondominant shutdown response, will present as moving toward the other to befriend and tend, and bracing and tension within the muscles due to the presence of the increased stress hormones adrenaline and cortisol. Other characteristics include heightened scanning of the environment and other nervous systems through sight and sound to predict potential threat. Forced and dramatic expressions of welcome, like smiling and laughing. Increased heart rate, respiration, blood pressure, and stimulation of sweat glands. Relaxation of the bladder. Inhibition or slowing down of the reproductive system, immune system, digestive system, and insulin activity. Nausea or butterflies as blood motility is directed away from the stomach and to your muscles and limbs for action-taking. Lightheaded or dizzy as a result of faster breathing.

Disorder or Response?

Common diagnosis (or misdiagnosis): dependent personality disorder, codependency, social anxiety disorder, or avoidant personality disorder.

When I Was in the Fawn State

My dominant survival response is flight, so it's no surprise that my second-most-visited survival response is fawn, which is a blend of flight and shutdown. Flight was the armor I wore to survive from my own discomfort; fawn was the armor I wore to survive others. Fawn is a protective pattern often developed in childhood when a caregiver was neglectful, abusive, or unpredictable—and is often centered in a deep fear of abandonment, rejection, or harm.

This abandonment wound has roots that date back to my time in the womb, when as an infant I lacked the connection and secure attachment needed from my caregiver to feel safe and regulated. My earliest years put me on a collision course for a lifetime of appeasement, abandonment of self, and codependency. From being the serial monogamist who jumped from one boyfriend who needed fixing to the next (until I met my husband in 2012), to subconsciously attracting people in my personal and professional life whose dominating fight response would keep me in my comfortable submissiveness (until I came into a space of healthy aggression and boundary setting), to forgoing confrontation and conflict at every turn while being the agreeable "pushover," fawn was my reliable crutch in relationships. Ultimately, it was through embodying my power and my sense of self that I was able to release the chronic chains of fawn.

5. Functional Freeze

Functional freeze is the state of autopilot and functional numbness. It's a blended state of both our dominant dorsal shutdown response and our nondominant sympathetic flight response, whereby we are mobilized in our day-to-day life while also disconnected and dissociated from our somatic experience—emotion, feeling, and sensation. It differs from our dorsal shutdown response in that we are not immobilized, shut down, depressed, and isolated (withdrawn in our turtle shell). And it differs from our blended freeze response in that we are not stuck in immobilizing shock (deer in the headlights). Instead, we are like the Tin Man, functioning yet emotionless and unable to feel or express what feels bad or even good.

Behavior Characteristics

Here, you are disconnected and detached from your body and often dissociated. Emotions are suppressed and, therefore, flat, numb, and unavailable to you. Like the "walking wounded," you go through the motions and seem to be unfazed by either good or bad experiences in your daily life. You're externally oriented. Disconnected from yourself, you tend to blend in with the world around you as you "just go with the flow." Because you have suppressed your feelings, you often lack the necessary charge and emotion to take offense or protect yourself—like anger, for example—creating an environment prone to abuse and limited boundaries. You often just take whatever life throws at you, adapting like a chameleon to survive whatever challenges you face.

What You'll Hear (Similar to Shutdown)

"That's just life."
 "I don't feel anything."
 "It doesn't matter to me."
 "Let's just move on."

How It Shows Up in Relationships

A communication style that often presents as little to no expression of emotion. You're neutral in all scenarios. You're agreeable and go with the flow of what the other person prefers because you're disconnected from yourself and your own desires. This can come across as acting like you're disinterested, distant, or don't care. You find it difficult to show connection as well as feelings of offense or hurt. You're here but not here in the relationship.

JENNIFER'S STORY

I was in a relationship for twenty-five years that was marred by a significant amount of infidelity, including the birth of someone else's child. I struggled but stayed in the marriage for years to prioritize what I believed to be the best path for my two children. Yet over time, I found myself completely lost in the turmoil. I now know that at the root of this "stuckness" was a years-long functional freeze that left me vulnerable to his emotional and eventually physical abuse.

I remember the turning point. I had been out with a girlfriend one night at a concert and had lost my phone. When I got home my husband was outside pacing like a tiger. He banged on the car as I pulled into the garage. Terrified, I hesitantly got out of the car. What would follow would be the worst physical experience I'd ever had. The next morning, I was bruised and sore, yet the first thought running through my head was, *Well, I deserved that.* The words froze me in my tracks. It was such a startling thought and one that I recognized was wrong. *Of course* I didn't deserve that.

Although it took another full year to completely disengage, that was the start of the separation from my husband. But life wasn't done testing me. Soon after the split, I was diagnosed with cancer. I once again felt stuck and unable to move forward. It was without a doubt the hardest season of my life. On top of that, any text, phone call, or communication from my husband would set me even farther back. I spent months and months in that hopeless state.

I found Brittany when I needed her the most. I'd been listening to a dating podcast with some friends as a fun distraction, and the hosts had Brittany Piper on as a guest speaker. While I found her story incredibly moving, what resonated with me wasn't the moment of impact in relation to her traumas, but the devastating aftermath. There was something in her experience that was ringing true for me—that trauma wasn't just about a specific life experience but the ongoing repercussions and survival responses that we don't even recognize are there.

I started following Brittany on Instagram, consuming her relatable and educational content on trauma. She was sharing information about somatic healing, the nervous system, and its connection to trauma—all of which was new to me. When she mentioned her Body-First Healing Program, I looked it up and started to fill out the application but ultimately chickened out. Looking back now, I can recognize again the ways in which my functional freeze ruled over my life. The *I have to do this! Oh wait, I can't* feeling was too much to override.

So I continued to follow Brittany on social media and decided to coach myself instead. My career is in learning and development, whereby I provide coaching in my day job, so I figured I could try my techniques on myself. It didn't take long to realize it doesn't work the same way. The truth was, I was not in a better place at all. In fact, I was still really stuck. That's when I decided to see if maybe Brittany could help.

In my first session with Brittany, she asked me what I hoped to achieve in the program and in our work together. I told her I wanted the anxious butterflies in my stomach to go away and that I felt stuck in every aspect of my life.

"Well," she told me, "I can't promise you these feelings or triggers will ever completely go away, but what we can do is work on finding more capacity to experience them and even possibly move through them." And that's exactly what happened. Although I didn't yet understand how Somatic Experiencing works, Brittany gave me the tools and approaches to learn how my unique nervous system was informing my everyday reactions, behaviors, emotions, and thoughts.

At the time I had been such a believer that I could think my way through any situation, be logical and rational—the typical assumption that the body itself isn't rational or isn't the site of knowing. I had to start small within my own somatic healing journey, trying different grounding techniques for resourcing for instance, until I eventually found one or two that worked best. When I focused on my body, I was able to support myself through challenges and discomfort with the tools Brittany gave me.

I also learned that somatic healing is a process; there are inevitable highs and lows that you go through in life, and you can get stuck again. This happened a few months ago when something didn't happen the way I'd hoped and it triggered me back into a functional freeze. When this happens, I can offer myself a lot more grace and understanding. Additionally, I can go right back to my set of tools to process it head-on so I can move back into healthy functioning much quicker. I can also use the same tools with my kids. They were teens when my husband and I separated, and they, too, struggled with trying to figure out what had happened to our family. Although we didn't know we had these built-in tools back then, I now can use somatic techniques with my kids, who are more like young adults today, to help them work through their challenges.

Most of all along this journey, I've had to learn to love *her* (myself) again. For so long I had put such a premium on my brain while completely disregarding my body, a body that had been hurt terribly in so many ways, not just physically but also emotionally. I started loving *her*, truly caring for my body and not seeing it as my enemy or something to tame or control. I grew up as a serious athlete and had been a distance runner in college. I had spent many years of my life controlling and monitoring everything I ate and how I worked out. On the one hand I had a body that enabled me to run as fast as I could, but it also was a body I abandoned when I was constantly restricting calories and abusing alcohol to just disappear into my freeze.

Through working with Brittany, I came to see that there is no separate mind or body. By starting small and really learning to love *her*, and by understanding that being allowed to feel isn't a battle or a fight, my life has become so much better. I realized I was not broken and didn't need to be fixed. Even more, when I care for *her*, she does really great things.

How You Carry It in Your Body

The hallmarks of a blended functional freeze response carries with it disconnection from one's body and possible dissociation, while still having access to the mobilizing hormones of our sympathetic response. This dominant shutdown response, blended with a nondominant fight-or-flight response, will present as a neutral or slouched spine along with periods of loose and then bracing muscles. Other characteristics include: decreased scanning and awareness of threat, instead presenting as a downward gaze or blank stare. Sensory information goes offline (halting at the thalamus) as endorphins release to numb pain and dynorphins release, allowing you to dissociate from your inner and external world. Decreased heart rate, respiration, blood pressure, and body temperature. Pale and cold skin and limbs as blood motility moves to the core to keep vital organs supported for "hibernation." Inhibition or slowing down of the reproductive system and immune system.

Disorder or Response?

Common diagnosis (or misdiagnosis): schizoid personality disorder, or autism spectrum disorder.

When I Was in the Functional Freeze State

Much of my early speaking career was spent presenting on stages where I felt completely detached from my body. "Robotic," I would critique myself. The first few years, I remember being confused about why I felt little to nothing when I'd share some of the most difficult parts of my life. Of course, knowing what I know now, it makes a lot of sense. It was my biology's and physiology's brilliant way of protecting me from what it perceived was too much.

Determined to "get better" and embody my words and experiences, I began working with a speaking coach and even joined a public speaking club (Toastmasters International) to grow my skills. Of course, it wasn't until I began my somatic healing journey that my speaking really changed, allowing me to be more expressive through my words and even welcoming moments for tears when they would come up.

This wasn't the only time in my life that I became stuck in a long functional freeze. I think back to the season of my life when the trial was happening. How numb I felt during that two-year period, unless I was drinking—when the suppressed rage would come barreling out. But during that time, I was often told by those around me that I was "so strong" and handling the whole thing "so well."

Going through the motions as a way to suppress my feelings was my only way of surviving during that time. I remember even during the trial, taking the witness stand and feeling absolutely nothing as I stared at my perpetrator from across the courtroom. By that point I was hardened and numb. Following the trial, I gave an interview to one of the local news crews covering the case. I can still recall sitting with my parents that night, watching the TV as the news anchors discussed the trial among themselves. One anchor stated, "I was telling Dave [his co-anchor] earlier, that in twenty years of covering court trials, I don't believe I've ever seen a rape victim who was this *poised*, this *composed*, who was able to look her rapist in the eye and say, 'You did this, and you're going to pay.'"

I believe so many of us today, in this modern and detached world we live in, are the walking wounded. We're functioning day-to-day on autopilot, seemingly calm and collected. Yet we've become completely disconnected from our true nature, from the very real and productive emotions and feelings that are attempting to keep us in a place of presence and expression and restoration.

YOUR HOME AWAY FROM HOME

Begin to think of your *stuck personality* as your home away from home. Your true home is in ventral, at the top of the Polyvagal Ladder. This is where you feel safe and connected—to self, the world, and to others. Although the aim is to get you unstuck, you'll naturally find that you'll still gravitate toward that armor in the future as your dominant protective state. And remember, that's okay. Regulation doesn't mean always being at the top of the ladder; it means being able to move up and down the ladder with ease and flexibility, and without getting stuck.

THE POLYVAGAL PERSONAL PROFILE MAP

Based on the Polyvagal Theory framework, Stephen Porges and Deb Dana developed the Personal Profile Map, which begins the skill of noticing and naming—where you notice a certain emotion, thought, behavior, and somatic cue and can name which state you're in based on that information. This is an important first step in being able to learn the language of your nervous system and accurately move yourself out of dysregulation. Before moving on to the core wound process in the next section of this chapter, I invite you to complete your own Personal Profile Map on page 273 in Appendix A.

Where Your Armor Originated: Your Core Wounds

My hands gripped the steering wheel as tears streamed down my face. My shoulders and chest shuddered as I gasped for breath through the sobbing. It was 2022, and I was on my way to the airport, leaving behind my husband and two-year-old son for a quick one-night work trip from Dallas to San Francisco, where I was going to be speaking at Sonoma State University. And here I was again, a blubbering mess. These panic attacks were a new occurrence for me, beginning shortly after Noah was born and showing up whenever I had to travel away from him. I found their presence quite perplexing because I had spent most of my career traveling the globe, separated for months at a time from the people I loved, without ever experiencing much distress.

These emotionally charged reactions were so intense that I had been having very serious conversations with my husband and booking agent about leaving the speaking profession so I didn't have to travel away from home. This was saying a lot, because speaking had always been a lifeline for me, a passion I'd never dreamed of walking away from. I had gotten so accustomed to these panic attacks that I would strategically plan my trips around them. I learned to avoid putting on makeup until I arrived at my destination; otherwise, my tears would smear it all away. I always wore a jacket or sweater with a hood so I could hide my puffy eyes in the airport. I learned to always book the first flight out so I could cry on the plane in the pitch black of the morning without anyone seeing me.

However, little did I know that this trip would bring with it what all the others before hadn't—clarity. I pulled into the Terminal A parking garage and quickly found a discreet parking spot nestled among a sea of cars. With plenty of time to spare before my plane boarded, I laid back my seat and curled into a ball, allowing the tears to continue. The next thing I knew, the nostalgic and gentle guitar riff from the song "I Hope You Dance" by Lee Ann Womack began to play over the radio. In a split second, I was catapulted back to the year

2000. The blurred silhouette of my eleven-year-old self appeared in my mind, like I had stepped back into a vintage reel of my childhood. As if reliving a memory of someone else's life, I observed her as she sat on her bed with a gift from her mother in her hands: a lyrical and inspirational book called *I Hope You Dance*. It was a sentimental keepsake her mother had wanted her to have, to encourage her to "keep dancing, keep living, even when life is hard." The cinematic lens hovered closer, and I could now make out the details of her face: sadness, loneliness, and longing. She wanted her mom.

I clutched at my throbbing heart, similar to how I clutched at my heart during my somatic womb work session on the therapy table that I described in chapter 4. The puzzle pieces swirling in my mind began to fall gently into place. In the span of a few seconds, it all made so much sense. The worry and anxiety that was coming to the surface every time I'd leave Noah was a traumatic imprint from the past, one that was triggering the experience of my mother living and working in another state every Monday through Wednesday for eleven years of my upbringing. Never in my conscious mind had I given this experience any thought or conviction. Never once had it occurred to me that there was underlying discomfort or unprocessed pain. Yet here I was, and here she was. This was a younger part of me that I was emotionally regressing to in these moments of departure from my son. And although I consciously know it's not true, in her developing subconscious, this younger Brittany had perceived that her mother's absence meant that she was again abandoned, unlovable, and alone. Another layer of healing to be explored.

I landed in San Francisco a few hours later after an emotional yet therapeutic flight. I distinctly remember driving over the Golden Gate Bridge as I spoke to my mother through the rental car speaker, telling her openly about the epiphany that had just transpired that morning.

"I never realized it back then, but I know now that I guess I just really missed you," I shared through tears.

What followed was a loving and transparent dialogue from both sides. She met my heartache and grief with such tenderness and understanding—apologizing for her absence and providing further context about why she had made those difficult decisions. And that context allowed me in return to hold forgiveness and compassion and even appreciation for that version of her. Even more, following that trip, the panic attacks ceased and the angst of leaving my children behind softened. This anxiety, this armor that was pushing me to the brink of running away from a career that I loved so much, had finally been removed.

This is the story for many of us who travel the road of recovery. As we begin to lift the armor that has kept us so closed off from immense pain, we often find that our core wounds, although we assume to be more glaringly obvious, also can be more invisible to the eye. I had spent so many years of my healing focused on the more discernible trauma, like the loss of my brother and the assault, that I had completely overlooked some of the more chronic experiences that laid dormant in my body and mind.

This next section will help you explore those moments for yourself, allowing you access to what I call the "Three C Inquiry": curiosity, context, and compassion. As we become curious about our armor—our patterns of protection—we gain more context around where it originated. This context then gives us greater capacity for self-compassion rather than self-judgment or self-criticism.

In my case, instead of beating myself up for the few times I still experience anxiety when I travel or leading with the *Why am I like this?!* attitude, I can now offer myself compassion for that younger Brittany when she comes up. I can hold loving space for that younger part of me that's simply trying to protect me.

Before You Start Your Core Wounds Work

As we begin the work of core wounds, I invite to you to be gentle with yourself. Resource and titrate the experience as best you can, moving through just one protective pattern at a time and giving ample space in between—at least up to a week. The intimate self-inquiry of some of your most least-desired patterns can bring up difficult feelings, emotions, and memories. These are some of the loving reminders I often give myself and others when beginning this process:

1. Keep your resources close. Resource before sitting down to do a core wound, take a break to resource throughout if needed, and anchor yourself in a resource again at the end. This could be an object you hold dear, having a person or pet close by to co-regulate with, doing the reflection outside so you can orient with nature through your senses, etc.

   » Also read more about resourcing on page 202 in part II so you have plenty of knowledge at hand before you start.

2. Although difficult, and perhaps not yet possible, can you attempt to do the following?

   » Thank yourself for armoring up in the ways you needed to to survive.

   » Appreciate the time it took to recognize the battle was over.

   » Remember that you protected yourself in the only ways you knew how to at the time.

3. Take all the time you need. If it ever feels like too much, you can always come back to this process when you're ready.

Your Protective Patterns

Think of your armor as the protective patterns or management strategies that once served to keep you safe but now may be hindering or even harming you. Consider these the symptoms of unhealed trauma. Common protective patterns include people-pleasing, isolating, self-medicating, pushing away love, overeating or undereating, procrastinating, lashing out, giving up on your career, being codependent, pursuing abusive partners, and so much more. Believe it or not, at the time, these behaviors were created to help you survive what was too overwhelming. So how do you change?

Merely changing the behavior won't resolve or heal these patterns. We have to get to the root of the symptom. For instance, perhaps you drink too much alcohol to cope, so you stop drinking. But then three months later you're overusing your pain medication. We call this *symptom-substitution, symptom management,* or *behavior modification*—where you jump from one maladaptive protective pattern to the next because you haven't healed or processed the root cause, or the *core wound.* When unhealed, core wounds create patterns of behaviors, thoughts, emotions, and limiting beliefs that keep you stuck in the protective states of the past. These are the implicit reactions and behaviors you scrutinize yourself for but can't seem to stop doing them.

Think of Core Wounds as an Onion with Many Layers

An onion is a common metaphor used in healing. And in this case, we can use it for understanding core wounds.

At the core of the onion is a trauma or experience, which creates the following layers from the inside out:

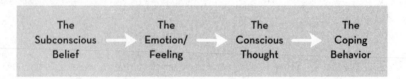

The Subconscious Belief → The Emotion/Feeling → The Conscious Thought → The Coping Behavior

It also can be illustrated like this:

- **Core wound:** Your trauma, which can be multiple events or experiences.
- **Limiting belief (subconscious):** Your core wound produces a subconscious belief about yourself, others, or the world.
- **Emotion:** That limiting (subconscious) belief creates an emotion that you feel in your body.

- **Thought (conscious):** That emotion creates a conscious thought (or story) in your mind.
- **Coping behavior:** That conscious thought (or story) produces an impulsive behavior.

Here are two things to note: First, the outside layer of the onion is your coping behavior—it's what everyone else sees on the surface. Second, your conscious thoughts sometimes differ from your subconscious beliefs. In other words, you don't always believe what you think or think what you believe. For example, subconsciously you may believe you'll always fail, yet your conscious mind tells you you're capable of anything—so you show up with confidence on the outside yet always "sabotage" (protect) in the end because your subconscious beliefs (guided by the ancient impulse of the nervous system) will always reign supreme.

Let's look at a quick example of the full onion to illustrate these points. If your core wound was being neglected as a child, it would then create a subconscious limiting belief that you are unworthy of love, which then seeds the emotion of toxic shame, which then creates the thought that relationships are pointless, which then leads to the coping behavior of avoiding and abandoning relationships altogether.

Your Top Five Protective Patterns

What are the top five behaviors you do that help you cope but that you feel are no longer serving you? Consider these your management strategies. (Hint: You may have identified some of these behaviors in the Naming Your Reactions reflection at the end of chapter 4.) Write these protective patterns in order from most present in your life (#1) to least present in your life (#5):

1. _____

2. _____

3. _____

4. _____

5. _____

Now, with titration in mind, we're going to start with your least-present coping behavior, and we'll be adding it into the core wounds formula next. This should be the coping behavior that causes the least amount of disruption in your life. With this protective pattern in mind, think about a recent time (not trauma-related) that you were actually participating in this behavior. As an example, let's say that you isolate. As you reflect on that memory, let's put the action into a statement while continually adding the word *because*. We're going to keep adding the word *because* to each statement until we hit a dead end. A dead end occurs when we can't think of a next response, or when we start to move from beliefs or thoughts to *facts* or *experiences*.

Here is a typical isolating scenario:

I isolate *because* . . . I don't want people to see me.

I don't want people to see me *because* . . . I don't want to be judged.

I don't want to be judged *because* . . . my emotions are embarrassing.

My emotions are embarrassing *because* . . . showing emotions is a weakness.

Showing emotions is a weakness *because* . . . that's what I was taught and shown as a child.

That's what I was taught and shown as a child *because* . . .

We stop here, because we are now talking about a fact or experience and no longer stating a general thought or belief.

When we hit a dead end, we ask, "Around how old was I when I remember believing this?" (This references the last statement of thought or belief.) As you ask yourself this, you can start to recall your life around that time and the circumstances you were in. This will reveal to us our core wound.

Let's continue with the example:

How old was I when I remember believing this (showing emotions is a weakness)?

I remember around the age of six feeling like I had to keep in my emotions because my parents were going through a divorce and told me to "buck up" because they didn't have time for my issues. So when I had emotions, I would go to my room to process them alone or hold them in altogether. And now, when I have emotions as an adult, I isolate and do the same. Also, I had a partner who would pull away or become distant when I showed any emotion, which just reinforced to me that my emotions weren't acceptable.

Now that you have identified the core wound, the next step is to consolidate all your layers (statements) into the final main layers of the onion.

So far, we have identified the behavior, the core wound or original trauma (which could be one or multiple), and the subconscious limiting belief. The subconscious limiting belief is the deepest statement of thought or belief before hitting that dead end. In this case, it was "Showing emotions is a weakness." What we're missing now is the emotion and conscious thought.

Let's move next to the conscious thought. Looking at the remaining layers or statements from the lines above, ask yourself which story is most true or most prominent for you. In other words, which thought sticks out the most? In this example, let's say it's "I don't want people to see me." Lastly, in search for the emotion, we can simply get curious about what we're feeling right now as we explore this protective pattern and this memory. What comes up for you? In this scenario, we could assume it's shame or embarrassment. The final step is to plug in all of the layers:

- **Coping behavior:** *Isolate*

- **Thought:** *I don't want people to see me (and my emotions)*

- **Emotion:** *Shame/embarrassment*

- **Limiting belief:** *Emotions are a weakness (or unacceptable)*

- **Core wound:** *When I was six years old, I had to keep in my emotions because my parents were going through a divorce and told me to "buck up" because they didn't have time for my issues. So when I had emotions, I would go to my room to process them alone or hold them in altogether. And now, when I have emotions as an adult, I isolate and do the same. Also, I had a partner who would pull away or become distant when I showed any emotion, which just reinforced to me that my emotions weren't acceptable.*

To summarize the final core wound statement, it would read like this:

I isolate because I don't want people to see me (and my emotions). I don't want people to see my emotions because I believe emotions are a weakness (or unacceptable). And I was taught this when I was six years old when my parents were getting a divorce and dismissed and discouraged my emotions; I later also had a partner who did the same. When I isolate, I feel shame and embarrassment.

What does your final core wound statement say? Write this out and reflect. Do you have a different perspective now of this protective pattern? Does it provide you with clarity and understanding that this behavior makes *so much sense*, and that in fact, *you* make sense? The ways that you've had to survive should make sense as well. Now, the next time you experience this protective pattern, I invite you to follow the Three C Inquiry:

1. **Curious:** First, as you start to engage in the behavior, you can get *curious* about it. Begin to ask what stories and feelings you are experiencing as this impulse or reaction starts to come up for you. Then inquire about the evidence that can be found in this moment that confirms these thoughts, emotions, and beliefs.

   » As previously mentioned, a trigger (which can be seen as an emotional age regression) will tell us that *we're in danger now*, when it often means *we were in danger back then*. In this particular example, if you perhaps start to feel emotion and overwhelm when with your kids and find yourself leaning into the impulse to isolate and go to your bedroom, you could pause (which will take practice!) and ask yourself, *What's the evidence in this moment that my feelings are viewed as a weakness or unacceptable to them?* When you get curious about these limiting stories and beliefs, you may find that they don't often ring true in your present circumstances.

2. **Context:** This inquiry leads you into the *context*, or the why behind your impulse, as you recognize it's just an old protective pattern being subconsciously triggered to come to your aid.

3. **Compassion:** This context grants you moments of *compassion* for yourself rather than self-judgment.

As we come into moments of acceptance for these impulses, we can begin to separate those younger protective parts from the present moment regulated parts. We can understand that the cloak of armor isn't always necessary, and that in moments of discomfort, we actually do have the capacity and resilience to have a different experience. That, for instance, just maybe, in this scenario, your emotions will be accepted by your kids. And it's this new evidence that gives us what we can call a *disconfirming experience*—when we are not reinforcing our patterns of survival and instead are having new experiences that disconfirm that need to armor up.

This is the first step in creating a new dynamic in the way that you relate to your trauma. Core wounds work allows you to separate past from present and recognize that safety, connection, and resilience can indeed be experienced in the here and now. The next step on this journey will be to move from conscious awareness of our patterns to subconscious and somatic processing of these patterns. By doing so, we will gently allow the nervous system to process and complete in the here and now what was too overwhelming to deal with back then.

Practice: Noticing and Naming

Practice this once a day for the next week:

1. Notice your thoughts, feelings, and the way your body feels.
2. Name where you are on the Polyvagal Ladder. What state are you in?
3. Get curious. What does your nervous system want you to know in this moment? What's the story it's telling you?

CHAPTER 8

Healthy Aggression and Life Force: Rising into Your Power

Trauma disconnects us from ourselves because it would be too painful to feel so small.
—Peter Levine

Her tiny fingers clawed and scratched across my chest as I winced. Shia (pronounced *shy-uh*) was six months old, the same age Noah was when he started to exert his power, his healthy aggression, or what Peter Levine refers to as his *life force energy* and vitality. It's around this time in life that children begin to acquire strength in the body, in their physiology, and in their sense of self. This could be seen in the way Shia was now pushing and pulling her body across the floor; rising up and standing against objects; banging her toys loudly with all her might; pushing my face away when she was done with kisses; raising her voice into sporadic powerful screeches; and hitting, scratching, and kicking while nursing. She was powerful beyond doubt, and the baby bruises and cuts I carried proved that to be true.

It was in 1912 that Sigmund Freud labeled aggression as a physiological sense of "hostile or destructive behavior"—destructive of others and of self. So it should come as no surprise that through our conditioned lens of what's "proper" or "good" behavior in humans, some might view Shia's aggression as hostile and destructive, thereby labeling her a "difficult baby." Yet nature's blueprint provides that not only is this behavior normal, but it's also vital and necessary for her development. When we look to the natural world, ethologists have found that aggression in animals offers biological benefits for survival, such as securing and maintaining territory, food, and water; protecting the self, offspring, or the pack; and offering reproductive benefits as males fight for mates, with the strongest prevailing. As human animals, we rely on our healthy aggression and life force in similar ways: to set and maintain boundaries (our version of territory), to defend ourselves or others (our pack), to advocate for ourselves, to speak our truth (therefore attracting deeper and healthier connections), and to propel us in life.

It's this propulsion and power that allows us to move forward, to keep going, and to get what we need out of life. In fact, when we deconstruct the word *aggression*, we find that it comes from the Latin joining of *ad* and *gradi*, meaning "step at," which figuratively translates as "stepping toward something, to go." The French call it élan vital, the "vital force" or the "vital energy." And in yogic traditions, *prana* is a Sanskrit term that translates as "life force" or the "vital energy" that's carried through the breath, body, and greater world around us.

Without this life force energy—which is physiologically bound to healthy aggression and power—we become stuck, no longer propelled to participate in the meaningful lives we desire. Our aliveness dims. That's where many of us find ourselves today, armored up and disconnected from ourselves, therefore disconnecting us from our own life force. Instead, we stay locked inside cages of our own making, where suppression and survival rule over us. In the journey of somatic healing, we aim to come back into the body, back to the parts of us we've been homesick for. For it's in the body that we hold tremendous wisdom, not just for healing, but also for living. In this chapter, I'll expand on the topic of healthy aggression and life force—how it gets extinguished at an early age, how it gets taken from us, and how we can rise again in our power.

When Life Force Was Extinguished at an Early Age

Our brains decide how we should and shouldn't exist in the world from the age of infancy. Most of our habitual behaviors, impulses, and subconscious beliefs form within our first few years of life—before we can even think or talk. Our perception of self, our perception of others, and our perception of the world are all shaped in these foundational chapters. And the overall trajectory of whether we become wired for survival or wired for aliveness takes shape through these implicit and somatic experiences.

So how does our life force—our power, healthy aggression, and vitality—become stifled during this season of life? There are innumerable scenarios, but here are some of the most common:

- **Intergenerational trauma:** We can carry on inherited impulses and subconscious beliefs through our cells that dampen our healthy aggression or power, which are then solidified by our lived experience in childhood. For instance, we can see this in homes where the relationship to anger is one of avoidance. This looks like growing up in an environment where the caregivers avoid healthy aggression, boundary setting, or rupture and repair cycles (such as disagreements), leading the child to believe that healthy aggression isn't normal or acceptable. This also can be seen in children who come from families that have experienced social and systemic trauma generationally, whereby their ancestors were part of a marginalized group brought on by slavery, war, genocide, colonization, immigration, and more.

- **Trauma in utero:** Trauma in the womb can promote shutdown and dissociation within the child's biology, disrupting the development of healthy aggression. Examples of trauma in utero could include the mother's exposure to trauma or extreme stress; drugs or toxins in the womb; oxygen deprivation in utero or during birth; prematurity; or medical procedures during pregnancy, labor, or delivery.

- **Developmental trauma:** This can happen when the conditions necessary for the development of healthy resilience and regulation were interrupted or compromised. Examples of developmental trauma could include ongoing danger, abuse, or addictions in the environment; neglect; being unwanted; separation from the mother as an infant or newborn (interrupting bonding and attachment); recurrent mis-attunement by the caregiver; medical procedures in first year of life; mothers who are chronically anxious, distracted, depressed, or disconnected to self; exposure to caregivers who are unable to regulate themselves; death of a parent or twin as infant or child; siblings born close together; or divorce while young.

Here are some more subtle and everyday examples of our life force or healthy aggression and power being stifled from an early age:

- We are conditioned and wired to suppress our healthy aggression. Let's pretend for a moment that Shia's relentless scratching, kicking, and hitting while breastfeeding was *too much* for my nervous system. And that her aggression, in fact, triggered me to the point of dysregulation, every time. If so, I might respond by screaming at her (which might startle or frighten her) or by putting her down and walking away out of frustration (which would also frighten her). From this repeated experience, her young brain and nervous system would begin to create the subconscious belief that power, vitality, and healthy aggression aren't safe, that her authentic expression would be met with rejection, and that to stay attached and accepted into the tribe she would need to suppress that impulse when it arises. As this pattern would continue throughout her formative years, and my dysregulation showed itself any time she expressed healthy aggression, she'd become further and further detached from herself. Later in life Shia would carry on this implicit response, dampening and suppressing her sympathetic charge and healthy life force, eventually leading to a cascade of relational, mental, and physical health problems.

Thankfully, I know how to attune to Shia's healthy aggression. By guiding her into a blended state of play—which, as we have learned, mixes the mobilizing experience of sympathetic fight or flight and the safe and connected experience of ventral—she is able to lean into that power by experiencing it, expressing it, and strengthening it alongside me. I'll do this by pushing her little hands against mine when they aim for my face, by stretching her legs when they coil back to kick me, and by praising her for her strength, all with smiles and laughs that make her feel safe.

PERI-PERSONAL SPACE

In the early months of life, infants engage in frequent limb movements, initially driven by reflexes and later by self-initiation—part of their life force and power. These movements bring them into contact with their own bodies as well as the objects and people in their surroundings. Despite appearing simple, these early movements serve as a fundamental process for infants to explore and understand themselves and the world they inhabit. Establishing a sense of our body is essential for interacting effectively with our environment. This involves understanding the position, speed, and reach of our limbs as well as our body's spatial relationship with the world around us. Peri-personal space is the area surrounding our body up to where our limbs can reach—think of it as your personal bubble— and it plays a crucial role in this process. Recognizing the boundaries and extent of our peri-personal space is fundamental for navigating physical and relational interactions and everyday experiences.

- We are conditioned and wired to suppress our healthy aggression due to toxic shame. Levine often talks about the difference between healthy shame and toxic shame. In our early years, there's shame that's healthy and helpful and shame that's toxic and harmful. Healthy shame is when our caregivers provide guidance and stern boundaries from a place of love and connection. When talking to my three-year-old son, Noah, I might say sternly, "Noah, we don't play with sharp knives, that could hurt us. And Mom doesn't want you to get hurt. So I'm going to take away these knives, and I don't want you to play with these again, okay?" My approach and delivery are clear and connected. From this place, Noah senses safety and connection, thereby granting him access to his learning brain.

  Toxic shame on the other hand, might go like this: "Noah! What are you doing?! What is *wrong* with you?! Go to your room right now, and don't you ever touch those knives again!" This approach is not delivered from a place of safety and connection, activating his amygdala (fear center) and causing

Noah's developing thinking and learning brain to go offline. Not only did he learn nothing, but he was traumatized in the process, and then sent away to handle it on his own. Dr. Gabor Maté poignantly shares that "Children don't get traumatized because of hurt. Children get traumatized because they're alone with their hurt."[1] Over time, this parenting style of constant belittling, humiliating or degrading, and rejecting Noah would get into not only his psyche—causing him to internalize that he's the issue, he's inherently bad, or that something is wrong with him—but also his cells and his physiology. This leads to the creation of a chronic environment of survival and illness.

Later in life, Noah would walk on eggshells in his relationships, learning that it's safer to suppress his authentic self, his life force, than to risk being humiliated or shamed again. He would operate from a place of suppression and disconnection, withdrawn from himself and stuck in a chronic cycle of functional freeze or shutdown. He would subconsciously associate physiological activation with threat (heat, higher heart rate, bracing and mobilizing of muscles, alertness). Anytime he would feel a sympathetic charge in his body, whether healthy or unhealthy (aggression, play, excitement, offense, drive, productivity, fear, frustration), he would autonomically shut it down. He'd be confused about why he procrastinates all the time, why he isolates, and why he feels so withdrawn. What Noah couldn't realize is that the antidote and healing medicine to toxic shame is healthy aggression—the one thing he's been rejecting. Instead of being shutdown, collapsed, and hidden away, he must learn to slowly reconnect with his life force so he can rise in his innate power. Shame speaks the story of "I am bad." Healthy aggression speaks the story of "I am powerful."

When Life Force Is Taken from Us Later

There are moments in our lives that, although they are fleeting, can leave a crater of destruction in their wake. A hole so big that life doesn't look, feel, or seem the same anymore. It's in these experiences that the *too much, too fast,* or *too soon* of adversity can rob us of our vitality, power, and life force, leaving us in a chronic state of shock, dissociation, or shutdown. From this place of disconnection, the rigorous climb out of this crater feels impossible, so why even try?

So how does our life force—our power, healthy aggression, and vitality—become stifled during later seasons of life? There are innumerable scenarios, but here are some of the most common:

- **Shock trauma:** These are the moments that overwhelm our physiology's capacity to cope. This is anything that feels like too much, too fast, or too soon. Some examples could be situations that compromise breathing (near drowning, suffocation, choking), serious asthma or high fever as a child, medical or surgical trauma, sexual assault or abuse, acts of violence, war, natural disasters, hallucinations or other intense drug experiences, motor vehicle accidents, physical injury, sudden loss of a loved one, near-death experiences, combat exposure, inescapable attack, and more.

- **Boundary rupture:** Boundaries enable us to set limits with others. They're where your body or yourself ends and someone else begins. Like your nervous system, your boundaries are unique to you, and when they're crossed, it's your healthy aggression and life force that asserts them. Any kind of violation of your boundaries is called a "boundary rupture." Most traumatic events involve a boundary rupture of some kind, including sexual, physical, emotional, energetic or spiritual, collective (experienced as part of a group), or informational (like the media). Boundary ruptures can have long-standing effects on our sense of self and life force, our connection with others, our perception of the world around us, and our capacity for accurate judgment in future boundary-setting.

For instance, as a result of a boundary rupture, our boundaries can either become *weak*, whereby we let everyone and everything in; *rigid*, whereby we let no one and nothing in; or *leaky*, whereby we spill out onto everyone and everything around us with little to no awareness of the impact.

- **Medical conditions:** A sudden medical diagnosis can induce a state of shock and functional freeze within the nervous system, shutting down our vital life force. The suddenness of such events often leaves us feeling powerless and vulnerable, exacerbating the trauma further. The subsequent stress, uncertainty, and physical discomfort associated with managing the medical condition can then trigger the release of increasing stress hormones, altering neural pathways, further heightening our need for survival, and pulling us farther away from vitality. Conditions could include chronic illnesses, neurological disorders, autoimmune diseases, cardiovascular conditions, cancer, and more.

BOUNDARY RUPTURES AND SENSORY SYMPTOMS

Any sensory channel can become increasingly sensitive or unavailable if a previous boundary rupture hasn't yet been repaired through the body. For instance, you might find yourself overly sensitive to light or to being touched or easily startled by loud sounds. Or, in contrast, you might find that your senses have become completely absent, like the resistance to looking in a certain direction or being deaf to certain sounds. Many of the tsunami victims in Indonesia, as an example, became temporarily blind because what they saw and endured was such an over-stimulus and intense trauma (too much, too fast, too soon). Fortunately, a team of Somatic Experiencing Practitioners arrived and provided somatic support, and most of the sufferers regained their eyesight. When you begin to use the somatic tools in chapter 10, peri-personal boundary exercises will allow you to feel into your "personal bubble" and notice which parts of your body or the space around you feel ruptured or strong.

The Chronic Illness Epidemic

In the intricate web of chronic illness, trauma often acts as both a catalyst and a consequence, perpetuating a relentless cycle of suffering. At its core, trauma can trigger physiological body-wide responses that exacerbate existing health conditions or pave the way for new ones to emerge. When it is stuck in the vortex of trauma, the body's primary goal is survival—weakening the immune defenses, increasing tension and inflammation, and leaving you vulnerable to illness. Over time, these bracing patterns within the viscera, muscles, and fascia begin to wear on the body, replacing ease and regulation with "dis-ease" and later disease and dysregulation.

Conversely, the burden of chronic illness itself can be traumatizing, robbing individuals of their sense of control, identity, and life force. This ongoing struggle can further amplify feelings of helplessness, isolation, and despair, perpetuating the cycle of trauma and illness. Breaking free requires body-based interventions that address both the physical manifestations of illness and the underlying emotional scars of trauma.

By this stage of our understanding that trauma requires a body-first approach, it should come as no surprise that a large majority of my clients in the Body-First Healing Program have some form of chronic illness or syndrome. In the somatic and nervous system healing space, this makes sense. Here's the potential path of chronic illness to illustrate why:

1. Adverse childhood experiences wire the developing nervous system to go into survival mode more easily.
2. Protective patterns and coping behaviors become set in place, further moving the nervous system into activation, alarm, and tension within the body.
3. Health challenges beginning from a young age can increase activation in the nervous system and amygdala activity in the brain, leading to deeper bracing within the muscles and viscera, catastrophizing, and, therefore, heightened pain.
4. Daily stress and major life changes in adulthood overwhelm an already fragile nervous system, worsening tension and physical symptoms into chronic form.
5. The brain becomes even more protective, as its attentional fear networks now become symptom-seeking to protect against the threat, creating again even more stress, tension, and heightened pain.
6. As physical symptoms become unbearable, daily life routines that bring about relief and the release of the pleasure-producing hormones become inaccessible (movement, connection with others, structure).

Too often I witness clients who are battling chronic conditions get wrapped up in a battle against themselves. They constantly self-judge when flare-ups or pain come back, leading to shame spirals, frustration, and a feeling of urgency to fix themselves. These are pathways that are familiar, patterns of suppression and self-shaming that kept them out of their life force and power, which perhaps was a necessary survival strategy in their formative years. But the internal belittling and obsession with fixing ourselves can make us even more sick because the very thing we're attempting to fight against—the body—is actually the one life force that can heal us the most. Unfortunately, what we resist will just persist.

Thankfully, there can be a path out of chronic illness. Through self-awareness and somatic healing, you can begin to come back into the vitality of life. From a place of self-awareness, the Three C Inquiry can help you shift these patterns and rewire neural pathways toward curiosity, context, and compassion. When we consider our symptoms with the Three C Inquiry in hand, we begin to move away from the *negative feeling we have about the feeling*, such as fear or criticism, and can start to dampen the alarm system that's creating heightened symptoms and responses.

With a somatic approach, you can address the emotional distress that creates another layer of dysregulation around the symptom. For instance, I had a client who had suffered for years from chronic migraines and, therefore, had created attentional networks that were constantly orienting to the smallest shifts that the migraine was coming. This fear around her chronic migraines created management strategies aimed at staying home to avoid bright light that seemed to activate the migraine. In this case, we began by differentiating between "How do you feel the pain?" and "How do you feel the *fear of the pain?*" By working with the fear first, we were able to discharge or decrease some of the overall activation, which in turn decreased the symptoms themselves.

By focusing less on the reduction of pain and more on how you relate to the pain, as well as building the capacity to be with what feels good and supportive, you can begin to heal. It is worth noting that chronic conditions can often begin in our earliest years due to trauma and, therefore, can take time to heal. This long and drawn-out process then creates deeper urgency and desperation to "fix" the issue, which can be subconsciously experienced all the way into the deepest layers of our viscera. You might find yourself thinking or saying, "I can't live like this anymore," "I have to get my life back," or "My body has betrayed me." Instead, I often encourage my clients to think about symptom elimination as a potential, whereby we first focus on step number one, which is granting them a better quality of life. It's from here that we slowly and gently bring presence into what is, without the need to fix, "solution-ize," or change anything about it.

Rising Again

Much of the mainstream nervous system chatter shines a spotlight on calming down, expressing our emotions, being present, and anchoring into regulation. But nervous system regulation isn't just about grounding into safety and releasing trauma from the past; it's also about re-creating the connections to our innate power and healthy aggression—your life force, in other words. This is the ultimate goal in somatic work: to bring you back into your body, which is the entry point and link to aliveness and self-healing.

Recently, my grandmother and I discussed the patterns of illness that plagued the women in our family, dating back five generations: congestive heart failure, breast cancer, strokes, atrial fibrillation, stress ulcers, and diabetes, just to name a few. I now see that these illnesses were a result of the somatic wear and tear of unhealed trauma passed down the line, the deeply ingrained beliefs that we had to muscle through, and the difficult experiences and feelings we had to suppress, all while standing alone. This pattern, a bracing and constriction to *keep it all contained and together,* created toxic internal environments that kept us prone to illness and made healing more difficult, too.

It was during this conversation that my grandmother told me about the time when she began to have more serious health problems, including multiple mini-strokes. "I was searching for all the answers outside of myself to heal," she told me. In essence, she was still running away from herself. She traveled the globe, living in ashrams, and even rented a home on the beach to live by herself for a year. But when she had a massive stroke in 1999, which left her partially paralyzed and housebound when she was only fifty-nine, she "was forced to stop searching outside of myself, and finally look within" and ultimately came home to herself. Still physically disabled and unable to leave the house today, she has said that her stroke was the greatest thing that happened to her. Even with her physical difficulties, her life has taken on a new meaning and a new feeling of empowerment and vitality.

Working with Your Life Force, Not Against It

I often look back on Noah's birth with sorrow. He was born in 2020, at a small birthing center in Fort Worth, Texas. It was at the height of the pandemic, so much of my pregnancy had been spent in quarantine with my husband. We took walks when we could, ate healthy meals, did in-home workouts, and dove deep into our virtual natural birthing classes. Although I thought I was prepared for an unmedicated birth, it turned out that my body didn't *feel* ready and fought me the entire way—all thirty-six hours of active labor.

Looking back now, I know exactly why Noah's birth turned out the way it did. I had become accustomed to being dissociated from parts of my body that experienced trauma, in particular my pelvic floor. When the contractions and sensations emerged in labor, crashing through like tidal waves that I couldn't possibly numb, I impulsively fought and braced against them, not allowing my pelvic floor muscles to relax so my baby could pass through. I was at war with my body and its innate ability to deliver my baby to me. I resisted my primal life force because I feared it. And the more I feared my body, the more activated my nervous system became, which meant the more stress hormones that coursed through my body, which meant the more tense I became, which meant the more pain I would experience . . . and the cycle would repeat. Throughout the entirety of my labor, I clung to my husband and midwives for support, not trusting I could do it on my own. It was a vicious, suffocating, and traumatizing experience I wasn't prepared for, one that left me feeling completely *disempowered*.

When I became pregnant with Shia three years later, I was determined to have a different experience, yet also be open to whatever would naturally unfold. I started seeing a pelvic floor therapist and began to research physiological birth—learning how to work *with* the unique and natural hormones of the body that arise during the birthing process rather than fighting *against* them. It was also around this time that I discovered a birthing style called "empowered birth." The mission behind an empowered birth is to rewire the neural pathways underlying your fearful subconscious beliefs so you can foster a profound sense of trust in the body and its primal wisdom, thereby allowing you to get out of your own way.

Shia's birth in 2024 was a complete 180 compared to what I'd experienced with Noah. Instead of going into the birth fearing the process and resisting my body, I leaned into the sensations of both power and pain. This time I was attuned to the experience. Throughout the seven-hour home birth, I gently disappeared into myself, into my body, and into the bond between baby and mother. We rode the waves of life force steadily, breathing into its power and wisdom. Tears of love and gratitude flowed. I spent most of the birth in my own little bubble, and later my husband and team of midwives told me it was like I was transported into another world, a state of bliss and power. Now, when I look back at the few pictures taken from my husband's phone, I'm in awe of the loving and euphoric smile I have on my face, during what was likely the hardest moments. I was reconnecting with my body in the most profound way and allowing it to carry me through, and for that I was so appreciative. By tapping into my vitality, I was able to have a natural "empowered birth."

The next steps on this Body-First Healing Roadmap will guide you on the same path back to yourself, where you'll learn exactly how to experience and attune to your body, how to express it and expel what's stuck, and how to reconnect to your own powerful life force.

Exercise: The Polyvagal Regulating Resources Map

Based on the Polyvagal Theory framework, Stephen Porges and Deb Dana developed the Regulating Resources Map. As you know, you naturally move up and down the Polyvagal Ladder all day, every day. This map identifies what you need to do to self-regulate or co-regulate and help you track your steps. I invite you to complete your own map on page 275 in Appendix A.

PART II

Somatic Experiencing Roadmaps

CHAPTER 9

Somatic Experiencing Basics

There's what we know, and there's what we feel. And often, there's a mismatch between the two.

As in:

I *know* I need to set a boundary, but I *feel* afraid to do so.

Or:

I *know* I deserve better in this relationship, but the potential for loneliness *feels* worse.

As we've learned already, the primal and subconscious impulses of the body will almost always override the conscious thoughts in our mind.

Life becomes even more difficult when we've experienced trauma that keeps us stuck in protective patterns, guided by feelings of fear, anger, or helplessness—patterns that seem incongruent with how we envision the life we want. This is the differentiation that Somatic Experiencing brings. Through a body-first approach, we allow the body to experience small and tolerable moments of discomfort, widening our tolerance to be with what's *different*.

For example, imagine you get a text message from a family member who often needs your help, asking you for yet another favor. Instead of saying yes, even though you know your plate is full, you could instead pause and notice the sensations that accompany whatever fear you might have about saying no. Maybe it's the shallow breath as you read their text message. Perhaps it's your sweating hands, the bracing of your arm muscles, the collapse or slouching of your shoulders, or the pit in your stomach. As you take time to simply notice and observe those sensations, what might happen next? You don't need to make sense of them or even try to change them. Just take time to *experience* them, making space for the natural expression and expelling of stress hormones to follow.

Just as your body knows how to digest and metabolize food, it also knows how to metabolize and process emotions and sensations. It's important to note here that it takes the body an average of ninety seconds to move through a feeling. In this case, maybe as you read the text message, you take time to notice the sensations that arise—now your arms have an impulse to stretch up and out, expanding your chest as you take in a large inhale down through your belly and let out an even larger exhale. It feels like relief, followed perhaps by openness in your chest and now a rising of your shoulders and straightening of your spine. The pit in your stomach has dissipated. You feel like you're taking up more space now. You feel powerful and assertive— even your eyesight seems to have more clarity. You *feel different*. Less afraid and more courageous to say no.

It's these small somatic experiences, felt over and over, that begin to change the outdated protective patterns that are keeping you stuck in survival. And over time, you build new muscle memory.

This is a preview of what Somatic Experiencing looks and feels like. When we get out of our heads and allow the *natural experience* of the body to intentionally and intelligently guide us, subtle transformation and healing can begin to take place. Here, we can explore new feelings, new choices, and new outcomes. Somatic Experiencing aims to support us in experiencing, expressing, and integrating the needs of our body and physiology. We do this so that we can . . .

- Have a new emotional and somatic response to an experience that was historically met with protective patterns (like leaning into fight/power instead of habitually shutting down).

- Bring an experience that's keeping us *armored up* and stuck in self-protective patterns of the past to somatic completion (which I'll explain in this chapter).

- Create a greater capacity to attune to our bodies and be with all our experiences, both pleasant and unpleasant.

Ultimately, healing through Somatic Experiencing helps you reconnect with yourself—the natural rhythms and desires of your body, your innate resilience, and the built-in resources you already possess to be your own best healer. It supports you in rediscovering and reconnecting to who you were, before the trauma told you who to be.

The Building Blocks of Somatic Experiencing

In the following chapters, I'll gently guide you into the somatic process to help you slowly begin to remove the protective armor of the past. Before you dip your toes into the work, it's important that you understand the building blocks of Somatic Experiencing (developed by Dr. Peter Levine) and its core concepts, which I'll explain through one of my own somatic experiences. Keep in mind that you should explore deeper work with a qualified Somatic Experiencing Practitioner, but this chapter is a powerful guide to get you started. I've included a short glossary at the end of this chapter to summarize the terms you'll learn, and for you to use as a resource.

A Preview of Somatic Experiencing: Out of Your Head and into Your Body

As you may have gathered by now, my tendency to fawn, appease, and make myself agreeable was a protective pattern I learned early in life. Every assessment I've ever taken, including the Stuck Personality Nervous System Assessment I created at the Healing Hub, has resulted with fawning finishing at the top of the list. It makes sense really, given my attachment trauma and subsequent fear of abandonment. By growing up in a hostile environment where I learned to walk on eggshells, in a home where it felt like anger would erupt at any moment, I became exceptionally good at reading people, picking up on the subtlest cues of dysregulation and danger. When turbulence would occur, I learned to run, hide, or pacify as a way to avoid or calm the waters. At a very young age, I became a master at placating myself, and also my parents. I was often thrown in the middle of their explosive arguments, enlisted to take on the role of peacekeeper.

It was during this early, chronic exposure to chaos that I formed the instinctual belief that keeping the peace and suppressing my own power, wants, and needs meant staying safe. It was a brilliant management strategy, really, allowing me to avoid conflict or rejection. But over time, this deep desire to stay connected to others, no matter the personal sacrifice, created enormous disconnection from myself. It's this reflection that always brings me back to the quote by Brené Brown that states, "Fitting in is about assessing a situation and becoming who you need to be to be accepted. Belonging, on the other hand, doesn't require us to change who we are."[1] This chameleon strategy was an adaptive response that, over time, became maladaptive as I became increasingly tolerant and vulnerable to individuals who were exploitive, manipulative, and ultimately unsafe.

In addition, what I had always seen as my best trait—to trust in the good of people—at times had been my biggest downfall. Although I could *feel and sense* that my perpetrator, the man who needed a ride home, was unsafe, I decided to let him into my car anyway. Although I could *feel and sense* that some of my personal relationships were one-sided and depleting, I still gave and gave to those people. Although I could *feel and sense* that people in my work orbit had possible ulterior motives, I gave them the benefit of the doubt anyway. My husband would lovingly and jokingly call me a "pushover," encouraging me to "stick up for myself more," "choose myself for once," "stop putting others first," but that was a lot easier said than done. Perhaps it was that I truly did believe in the good in people, or perhaps I just wanted to prove my history wrong—that people could be reliable, safe, and trusted.

Over time, Somatic Experiencing helped me to break this pattern. Several years ago, I had to draw a stern boundary with an employee with whom I had regularly struggled to bring constructive guidance to, due to their combative nature. Although the tell-tale signs had long been there, it wasn't until after our professional relationship came to an end that I realized I had been working alongside a "victim narcissist"—a subtype of narcissist who consistently acts like the victim and refuses to accept responsibility for their actions when all other forms of manipulation, vengeance, dominance, or control have failed.

In the few occasions where I'd actually mustered the courage to approach this associate, they would respond to my gentle requests using manipulation tactics—whereby they would become emotionally distraught and defensive—finding some way to twist the truth and blame me, or others, for whatever small issue needed to be addressed. In the end, I'd always end up being the one to delusionally apologize.

Over the years, this person had learned exactly how to play off of my agreeable and empathetic nature. They knew I avoided conflict and often cowered at it. They knew I could be overly forgiving and tolerant of disrespect. And they knew that because I believed in the good in people, I would cater to their upset feelings over my own. So, I'd always walk away from those dialogues dismissing my initial grievances, flipping the responsibility on myself, and apologizing to keep their peace—at the expense of my own. Appeasing was my safeguard. *Note: if every time you confront someone about something and end up being the person apologizing or taking the responsibility, run.*

Yet one day, it came to my attention that this associate had done something so egregious, so deceptive, so devoid of integrity, and so exploitative that I couldn't not say something. Although the act in question was so shocking that I was advised to immediately terminate their employment, I made the choice to instead give them a written warning and the opportunity to explain their actions and make it right. However, in the same breath, I made myself a promise to cut ties if they responded with their typical manipulation and deflection.

So, I anticipated and prepared for the worst, yet hoped for the best. Unfortunately, the conversation went just as it always had—attempting to twist the truth (even though we had the hard facts that caught them in the act), defensiveness, tears, and playing the victim. Although it wasn't easy to do and it went against the instincts of my body to just tolerate the abuse, this time around I knew I had to choose myself for once.

I can vividly recall the somatic experience of what happened in my body before that Zoom meeting began.

The underpinnings and sensations of fear became palpable. My solar plexus (the area right at the top of my abdomen) turned electric and constricted. I felt an upward bracing and holding, as my breath, shoulders, and neck lifted—priming me for impact (or, in this case, the potential confrontation that was coming). Nausea was now making itself known, as well as the radiating heat in my hands and armpits. It was full-blown fear, adrenaline coursing from head to toe.

On the edge of overwhelm, I reached for the pencil holder on my desk, turning it upside down and emptying the contents into my hand. Four shimmering rocks rolled into my palm. My resources. These were stones I had collected from Avalanche Lake. My mind began to drift to one of my favorite places in the world—a glacial lake located in the higher alpine regions of Glacier National Park in Montana. You can access Avalanche Lake only after a steep yet breathtaking hike through a thick cedar and hemlock forest. The scenic payoff is at the end of the trail, where you find Avalanche Lake in all its natural glory. I had completed a number of sunrise hikes to Avalanche during my many trips to Glacier, and each time I'd pulled a beautiful stone from its frigid, placid, and transparently blue waters to remember the moment.

I could feel the coolness of the stones as I rolled them around in my palm now. A deep inhale suddenly followed. The parasympathetic brake pedal of my nervous system was instinctually coming to my aid, attempting to slow down me and my rapidly beating heart. I again brought my attention back to my inner world, tracking the bodily sensations I could identify, a practice known as interoception. This time I followed the experience with just one interoceptive cue, the tightening of my solar plexus. On a scale of one to ten, with ten being the most intense, this was about a five. I could handle that. I bowed my head and closed my eyes. I sat quietly and simply allowed myself to observe the sensation, not rushing to make it *go away*, not attempting to *fix it*, to *label it*, or to even *understand it*—that could come later. In this moment, I just wanted to attune to the sensation and allow it to be seen, heard, and held.

As I gave my attention to my solar plexus, the constriction began to feel tighter again, moving upward even farther and expanding into my diaphragm. It was suddenly harder to breathe. The bracing was now reaching a seven in intensity. I impulsively squeezed the rocks in my hand, feeling the jagged edges against my skin. My eyes followed as I squeezed them closed and bowed my head forward while placing my opposite hand on my knee, allowing my body to lean into the welcomed support. Another sudden inhale, this time deeper and more expanded. An image appeared in my mind of the weight machine with the pulley system at my gym. With my eyes still shut, I envisioned the weight being lifted up, as if the weight of this constriction was being released from my solar plexus and pulled upward.

My eyes opened suddenly. My spine straightened as I sat back up and let out an audible sigh. An immediate energetic release and charge coursed up and out of my body. It felt like pure and primal power. Before I knew it, my limbs mobilized me and I stood and began to pace around my office, shaking out my hands. The vocalizing continued, this time taking on the form of a guttural low growl, "Rarrrrrrr." I could feel the heat coursing out of my body as I clenched my fists. I was rising into my power, my healthy life force and aggression. As my breath began to soften, I sat back down and pulled my hand to my chest, placing it over my solar plexus, where expansion had now replaced the constriction. I felt open, confident, appreciative, and supported. My mind moved to meaning—*I am powerful, my boundaries are important, I am open to this experience, and I can handle whatever follows.*

This was the productive fight response I needed in order to set a boundary. Yet, in this relationship I'd been suppressing it with fear—fear of retaliation, fear of conflict, fear of disconnection. This healthy aggression was a necessary and healthy impulse I had thwarted over the years in most of my relationships. It was this suppression that allowed my fear of abandonment and rejection to overpower my desires to advocate for myself and caused chronic fawning.

But by choosing to attune to my body and be with what it was experiencing, rather than rushing to fix it or get out of what was happening (by avoiding the conversation or jumping ship), I had the opportunity to create new feelings, sensations, and experiences. I allowed the healthy aggression to stay. I didn't retreat and withdraw.

Instead I sat tall, firm, and courageous. Finally, I set the stern boundary this associate had benefitted from me not having for all those
years. That was the last day they were employed by me.

The Language of the Body: Interoception and SIBAM

French philosopher René Descartes famously declared, "I think, therefore I am." The path traditional therapy has taken may have changed
dramatically if we'd understood this truth instead: "I *feel*, therefore I
am." Conventional talk therapy is rooted in cognitive thinking, and
as a result, it can't release the trauma that lies trapped within the
body and nervous system. Instead, Somatic Experiencing helps you
have a dialogue with your body by tracking its sensations—a process,
as you just read, known as interoception.

So how do we begin to understand the language of our body and
physiology? Somatic Experiencing Practitioners employ Levine's SIBAM
(Sensation, Image, Behavior, Affect, Meaning) framework to help our
clients work toward fully *experiencing a feeling*. By embracing each element of the SIBAM model, we can better process emotions, sensations, and our experiences in a way that is gentle and affirming. Like
learning any new language, it feels foreign and difficult at first. But
over time, with practice and repetition, you can become fluent in the
dialogue you have with your nervous system. To support you in this
practice, I have included a vocabulary of sensations list, as well as an
emotion wheel, on the next and following page:

Vocabulary of Sensation

Use this vocabulary to expand the language of your body and nervous system.

Achy	Firm	Numb	Snug
Beating	Flowy	Obstructed	Sore
Blocked	Fluid	Open	Spacious
Buzzy	Flushed	Paralyzed	Spinning
Bubbling	Fluttering	Pointy	Stretched
Burning	Freezing	Pounding	Strong
Chilly	Frozen	Pressure	Stuffed
Choking	Gentle	Prickling	Stuffy
Closed	Glimmering	Pulsing	Sweaty
Compressed	Goosebumpy	Quaking	Swollen
Constricted	Gurgling	Queasy	Tender
Cool	Heavy	Quivery	Tense
Cozy	Hollow	Radiating	Throbbing
Cramping	Hot	Raw	Tightening
Crampy	Icy	Restricted	Tingling
Damp	Immobilized	Robust	Trembling
Dense	Jerky	Roomy	Unsteady
Dizzying	Jittery	Rough	Vibrant
Easy breathing	Jumbled	Rumbling	Vibrating
Effervescent	Jumpy	Scorching	Warm
Elastic	Light	Sealed	Watery
Electric	Lightheaded	Sensitive	Weak
Energized	Limp	Shaky	Weightless
Expanded	Loose	Sharp	Weighty
Fidgety	Nauseous	Shifting	Widening

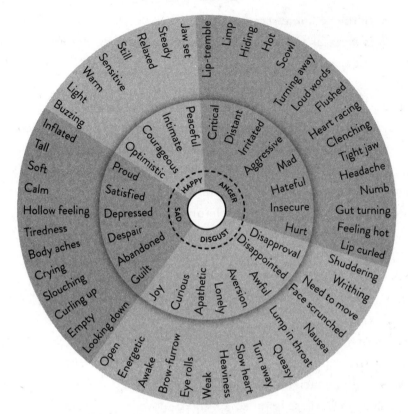

Adapted from the Emotion Sensation Wheel by Lindsay Braman

Let's look at each element, or channel, of SIBAM to support you in learning *how to feel a feeling*. I'll use the personal story I shared in this chapter to help guide you.

Sensation

Notice the bodily sensations associated with your experience. This could range from temperature changes to muscle tension. Instead of asking, *How am I feeling?* you ask, *What sensations am I noticing in my body right now?* To lead you into other channels, you might ask, *Is there a color or (Image) that goes with that sensation?*

- **In the personal story:** *I felt electric, constricted, nauseated, tension in my solar plexus, heat in my hands and armpits, expansion, calm, and open.*

Image

Imagery or memories can support the processing of an experience. These can include visualizations, dreams, symbols, memories, experiences, or places. For example, you might imagine a faucet or waterfall when you feel tears beginning to form or the color yellow when joy is present. To lead you into other channels, you might ask yourself, *As I imagine that, what (Sensation) happens inside my body?*

- **In the personal story:** *I imagined Avalanche Lake and a weight machine.*

Behavior

Notice the impulses or behaviors your body communicates, like gestures, sounds, facial expressions, or posture. When you can notice and slow down these impulses to micro-movements, they can lead to the completion of thwarted responses. For example, slowly straightening your spine into a confident posture can help if you feel like hiding in a collapsed posture. To lead you into other channels, you might ask, *Does this behavior have (Meaning)?* Or, *Does this behavior represent a certain emotion (Affect)?*

- **In the personal story:** *I experienced a rigid spine and a collapsed spine. I leaned my hand onto my knee for support, reached for my rocks, closed my eyes, squeezed the rocks, had sudden inhales, stood and paced, shook my hands out, clenched my fists, growled and vocalized, and put my hand to my chest.*

Affect (Emotion)

Identify the emotion you're experiencing. Tools like an emotion wheel can aid in this exploration, which you can see on page 195. To lead you into other channels, you might ask, *How do I feel the fear in my body (Sensation)?* or, *Is there a color or (Image) that goes with that emotion?*

- **In the personal story:** *I felt fear, power, aggression, confidence, appreciation, and supported.*

Meaning

Reflect on the meaning behind an experience. This will help you understand and integrate what's happening, and possibly even create new meaning around a previous limiting belief (as I did in the example above). To lead you into other channels, you might ask, *When I have that thought, what happens in my body (Sensation)?*

- **In the personal story:** *The first meaning that emerged was that rejection and confrontation were bound to happen. However, new meanings also emerged later: I am powerful, my boundaries are important, I am open to this experience, and I can handle whatever follows.*

When unresolved trauma resides within us, we often find that we lose access to some parts of the SIBAM model. For example, some people may have lots of emotions (Affect), but they cannot feel into their body (Sensation). Other people tend to lean into Meaning and Behavior, yet they cannot access their emotions (Affect).

The aim of the Somatic Experiencing approach is to integrate each piece so you don't just understand your experiences, but you also feel them.

BUILDING INTEROCEPTIVE AWARENESS

There are easy ways you can practice building your interoceptive awareness. Begin to track and note the sensations that arise when your body sends you signals that . . .

- You feel tired.
- You feel hungry.
- You need to go to the bathroom.
- You want to say yes.
- You want to say no.
- You feel safe.
- You want to set a boundary.

By bringing interoceptive awareness to the more neutral signals in your daily life, you can begin to create a deeper capacity to be with what's hard or uncomfortable.

Building Capacity

Somatic Experiencing aims to give you a greater capacity (or resilience) to tolerate being *in your body*, without becoming overwhelmed or shutting down. This means being with what feels good and what doesn't feel good. You build capacity by taking intentional time to slow down and move inward as you notice your interoceptive cues (sensations, feelings, and emotions) in the present moment. You first get comfortable being with the experience of the body before expressing or expelling what you couldn't express in the past.

Why is capacity important? When you don't have the capacity to contain your discomfort, it spills over, leaving you overwhelmed or helpless. In these moments, it's not that the emotion or discomfort was too big; it's that *your capacity was too small*. So in Somatic Experiencing, you learn to gently expand your capacity to experience your body without tipping over, before you can start the deeper trauma work. Let me use an analogy to illustrate this point.

Imagine that your capacity is like a hole you've dug in the sand, and discomfort is water that is poured into that hole. When your body and your nervous system have a decreased capacity to be with discomfort, your hole in the sand is small and shallow—therefore, more susceptible to potential flooding and overwhelm, because it's not big enough (resilient enough) to quickly absorb the water or discomfort. It's this limited capacity that often discourages you from even allowing in discomfort (the water). Instead, you suppress, avoid, or run from what doesn't feel good. In contrast, when your body and your nervous system have an expanded capacity to be with discomfort, your hole in the sand is wide and deep—it is resilient and not as easily overwhelmed by the waves of stress and discomfort that you experience day-to-day. That hole can contain and absorb the discomfort, without flooding.

Just as the body can naturally and innately process discomfort when given the chance, the hole in the sand can do the same over time. It will slowly and naturally absorb the water. And with practice, you will find that your capacity/resilience increases. When you gently allow water into the hole, the water will not just absorb into the sand, but over time, erosion will give way to a wider and deeper hole.

In the story earlier in this chapter, I allowed myself to be in my body as both the fear and the anger came up. Rather than trying to push it down, fix it, or make it go away, I simply slowed down and allowed myself to experience the natural waves of that arousal. Heat, clenching, and constriction eventually turned to expansion, softening, and a new sense of power and courage.

When you allow the wisdom of your body to guide you, it almost always brings you back to restoration. Growing your capacity—your resilience—is step one on the path to somatic healing.

Titration

Trauma happens fast; healing happens slow. In the wise words of Dr. Levine, the principle of "less is more, slower is better" guides us in a gentle process known as titration.

Titration is a term Levine borrowed from chemistry, whereby you combine two different solutions or compounds very slowly so they integrate in a way that avoids an intense chemical reaction. In fact, titration droppers have been designed to dispense only one drop at a time (quite the opposite from the volcano eruption experiments we had fun with in elementary school!).

This approach involves slowing down the therapeutic journey to counteract the overwhelming nature of trauma, which often manifests as *too much, too fast,* or *too soon.* Levine, knowing how sensitive a dysregulated nervous system is, found it paramount to create a method that would stretch the nervous system without further stressing it. Caught up in the trauma vortex of the past, titration helps us slow down the nervous system so we can catch up to the here and now.

So how does this impact somatic work? Here are two ways we use this concept:

- **Titrating or slowing down the *pace of a session*:** We invite clients to pause and move inward to track interoceptive experiences (sensations, feelings, and emotions).

- **Titrating or limiting the *content we explore in our sessions*:** In other words, we don't dive straight into the deepest and most intense traumas (the epicenter of the trauma vortex). Instead, we work the periphery and outer edges of challenging moments first. (I'll give you an example in a moment.)

When you combine these two ideas, it looks like this: we start our work with small fragments of mildly challenging experiences, pausing frequently to observe bodily sensations corresponding to the narrative. By allowing these sensations to unfold slowly and naturally, you can experience gradual moments of somatic completion, where the body can respond now in a way it couldn't respond back then. Examples include: saying no, defending ourselves, leaving or escaping, expressing our emotions, orienting to the oncoming threat, and more. In other words, by allowing for the slow and steady buildup of the previous survival charge (adrenaline and cortisol) to finally be accessed, experienced, and expelled, we can become *unstuck* from the self-protective armoring of the past.

When I began Somatic Experiencing after my assault, my practitioner helped me understand that I'd experienced a thwarted fight response during the event, and as a result, I had stored sympathetic activation in my system that needed to be discharged. But we didn't dive in headfirst. She began with a titrated approach by first guiding me in working through more manageable moments of anger. "Was there a moment recently that pissed you off?" she'd ask. As we worked through these smaller moments of anger, like when someone didn't listen to me, or when I received a rude email, I started to build a greater capacity to *contain and then expel* that activation (fight/healthy aggression) without getting overwhelmed. Over time, as I emptied the "pressure cooker" of fight from my system, I found that my irritability, frustration, and impulse to lash out became nearly nonexistent in my daily life.

A few final notes on titration: as a reminder, your nervous system prioritizes familiarity, even if it's not good for you. The formula of "same equals safe" still applies here. Therefore, you support your nervous system by titrating the healing process and allowing for slow and subtle healing and integration to take place. Often, I have clients who want to jump straight into change, transformation, and the deep end of healing. In Somatic Experiencing, we start in the shallow end, slowly making our way into deeper water.

Lastly, titration is instrumental in our expression as well. For instance, *forcing* a cathartic release of emotion or feeling before that unique nervous system is ready could further harm or re-traumatize that system—again, think *too fast, too soon, too much*. Instead, you want to follow the pace of your own unique system and allow it to *naturally release* and discharge in a way that feels tolerable. Now, this doesn't mean that a cathartic release won't naturally occur—raging, screaming, intense crying or shaking, for instance. That will depend on whether your nervous system has the capacity to contain that discomfort and experience.

Let's use anger as a quick example. I've had a large number of clients during the years who experienced physical or emotional abuse early in their life. As is often the case, their fight response, which was suppressed in those younger years because it would have been more dangerous for a small child to fight back, remained suppressed in adulthood. In working with these individuals, I would titrate the exposure to anger and healthy aggression as a way not to overwhelm the system or send them back into an intense trauma reenactment that they weren't prepared for. By introducing small and tolerable moments of the defensive fight response, we build the capacity to be with anger in a way that feels manageable. For instance, instead of immediately prompting my client to punch a pillow and scream, I instead might first invite them to slowly squeeze the pillow out of frustration and notice how that action lands in the body. This titrated approach allows the client to *be with the anger in the body*—metabolizing the anger and expanding their capacity—rather than jumping straight to a cathartic tool to quickly release, bulldoze through, or get rid of the anger. This titrated approach is a cornerstone of Somatic Experiencing, and it is paramount in preventing retraumatization.

Resources

As you learned at the beginning of this book, a resource is what you likely imagine it to be—anything internal or external that supports you in feeling a sense of okayness or betterness. This is what we call your "counter/healing vortex." Resources anchor you to a moment that feels either pleasant, grounded, safe, comfortable, supportive, present, or even just neutral. When you're actively engaging with your resources, you are *resourcing*.

Resourcing can be as simple as focusing on the support of the chair behind your back. Or it can be a memory, such as the sound of your children playing, or an observation you make in the moment, like the sight of the golden sunlight on the trees outside your window. In the story I shared earlier in this chapter, one of my resources was the rocks I've collected from Avalanche Lake.

Here are some basic resourcing techniques to explore:

1. **Internal tracking:** Is there a place of the body that feels more pleasant to be with?

2. **Grounding:** Can you feel the weight of your body in the seat or your feet stable on the ground?

3. **Visualization:** Can you paint a picture of an image, memory, or visualization that feels supportive?

4. **Orienting:** Slowly begin to explore the space around you with your senses, visual (sight), auditory (sound), tactile (touch), gustatory (taste), and olfactory (smell).

5. **Movement:** Large, gross motor movements could overwhelm the system, so inviting micro-movements is better, like feeling into a rhythm of the breath, gently sitting up straighter or leaning back, or slowly stretching—first with the fingers, then the hands, then the arms.

6. **Self-contact:** Is there a place in your body that would like some support or contact? As you offer your body some support, does it help?

7. **Co-regulation:** Is there a supportive other with whom you could connect for support? Or who you could imagine? This could even be a pet.

A general rule in somatic healing is that *you can only heal as much as you can resource.* To be able to go back and resolve unhealed trauma, you first need to build a sense of support and strength, inside and outside. This is the crucial first step in guiding and supporting your nervous system to come back to a state of ventral, to safety and connection. In the language of Polyvagal Theory, resources are the glimmers or neuroceptive cues of safety that your nervous system needs to promote regulation.

Every Somatic Experiencing session begins with identifying a resource and spending time with it so you can allow the nervous system to feel a sense of safety before moving into discomfort or activation. That might look like orienting to the room for a few minutes first, or simply leaning into co-regulation and chatting about a recent lighthearted funny moment. The possibilities are endless. Throughout the session, the practitioner guides you in oscillating or pendulating back and forth between this resource and the activating experience or discomfort that you're exploring. It's a very grounding kind of support, an anchor that pulls you back to the island of safety when overwhelm starts to pull you out to sea.

Pendulation

A healthy, regulated nervous system can move back and forth from a state of stress, or contraction, to one of calm, or expansion. We also think of these two opposing states as the trauma vortex and the healing/counter-vortex. One of the primary goals of Somatic Experiencing is to help you restore the ability to swing back and forth into both states, a natural biorhythm Peter Levine calls "pendulation."

Within a regulated nervous system, pendulation occurs moment to moment—we go back and forth from contraction to expansion throughout the day. Or, from the PVT perspective, when our nervous system is resilient and flexible, it can move up and down the Polyvagal Ladder with ease to adapt to what life throws at us.

I often describe pendulation by using an analogy of a grandfather clock. A healthy nervous system is like the pendulum in a clock, swaying from activation to deactivation, from fear to joy, from helpless to empowered—without becoming stuck at either end. A dysregulated nervous system, on the other hand, is like a broken grandfather clock. We're stuck at one end of the arc in the trauma vortex, where we remain armored up in a chronic state of contraction—either reenacting the turbulent tornado of the past, or shutting ourselves off completely in a state of freeze and suppression to avoid the suffering.

In Somatic Experiencing, we use pendulation to sway into both a resourced state and an activated state, moving back and forth between the two. By embracing resourced moments, we build confidence in our nervous system's ability to navigate challenges. This teaches our nervous system that it can experience stress and then come back to a state of calm or regulation, creating experiential evidence that will encourage our systems to no longer shy away from and avoid discomfort. Over time, and with practice, our nervous system becomes like the reliable pendulum of a grandfather clock swinging *automatically* on its own again, with even more force and resource, creating wider capacity to move through greater stress.

Somatic Completion and Discharging

As you know by now, Somatic Experiencing addresses the incomplete survival responses from the past we're still holding that create symptoms in the present day. The first step in doing this is to build the nervous system's capacity for this work. Then, in a moment of activation, a somatic practitioner might ask, "Is there something your body might want to do now, that it couldn't do back then?"

This is the process of somatic completion, of allowing your body and your nervous system to complete the thwarted protective or defensive responses of the past. It's in this moment of "completing the incomplete experience" that you are able to renegotiate the trauma by generating an active response where previously there was overwhelm and helplessness. These gentle and felt responses could show up as leaning forward in the seat, moving away by turning away, pushing away with limbs, pulling in and slouching to hide, straightening the spine, protecting or defending yourself or others, or restoring organic impulses. As you allow the opportunity in the present for these mobilizing responses to complete, the activation will begin to naturally discharge through shaking, tears, trembling, sweat, or heat.

Levine said he had an "epiphany moment" when creating Somatic Experiencing while working with a client named Nancy in 1969. In his book *Waking the Tiger: Healing Trauma*, he brought Nancy's story to life. Here is a brief summary:

Nancy was twenty-four years old when she first came to work with Levine and presented with a long list of physical and mental conditions she'd been battling since the age of four: fibromyalgia, irritable bowel syndrome, chronic fatigue, migraines, anxiety, panic attacks, and agoraphobia (fear of leaving her home). By the time she began her work with Levine, she had exhausted most medical options and had gotten no relief from her symptoms. In their first session, Levine worked with Nancy to help her relax into her body as a resource. During this process, they inadvertently uncovered the root of her symptoms: she'd had a tonsillectomy when she was very young, and before the surgery, the nurses and doctors held her down and administered ether, inducing in her sheer terror and shock. Levine theorized that Nancy's nervous system remained in that state of shock in the years that followed, wanting to escape but feeling trapped. During their session, Nancy was able to imagine running and fleeing from threat by visualizing a tiger ready to attack. After more than thirty minutes of this visualization, Nancy's body was able to muster the impulse to "run." At first, this visualization manifested as intense waves of shaking and trembling in her limbs and then the movements got softer. She finally had been able to tap into her body's innate defensive response, to do in the now what she couldn't do back then. This profound experience enabled her to renegotiate her trauma, allowing her to move from a feeling of overwhelmed helplessness to a sense of empowerment and agency. Nancy's symptoms, including the physical ailments that had imprisoned her for decades, resolved after only a few sessions. She later shared that she felt like she was "being held by a warm, tingling wave" during this process of somatic completion.

As Levine says, "Trauma resolved is a great gift, returning us to the natural world of ebb and flow, harmony, love, and compassion."

Putting It All Together: The Five Steps of Somatic Experiencing

By now, my hope is that you have a firm foundational understanding of the building blocks of Somatic Experiencing. When you put this understanding into a working framework, there are certain steps to take.

I again want to mention that when addressing trauma, it's important to have the help of a qualified Somatic Experiencing Practitioner, rather than try to do this work on your own. However, Somatic Experiencing also can help support through challenging everyday moments, as I'll illustrate in the example below.

As you follow these steps, the goal is to shift back and forth (or pendulate) from activation (the discomfort) to deactivation (your resources). In short form, this process can be summarized as *resource, experience it*, then *express it*, then *resource again*.

Here are the five steps:

1. **Resource:** Create a felt sense of safety (your supportive healing/counter-vortex).

2. **Pendulate:** Using titration, gently touch into the trauma vortex or discomfort by using interoception or SIBAM to notice how your body is experiencing this moment.

3. **Somatic completion:** Is there a *natural impulse* (don't force it!) to express or respond in a way you couldn't before?

4. **Discharge:** This will naturally follow completion. (You may feel tingling, shaking, or heat in your body, or cry, etc.)

5. **Resource:** Anchor back into your initial resource.

Here's an example:

Imagine that you have just arrived at a social gathering, and you are greeted by a group at the door. You're caught off guard, because one of the people in this group is someone who triggers you due to a previous experience of harm or hurt. Here is how you would use the five steps of somatic experiencing in this situation:

1. **Resource:**
   » If it feels like too much to be with this sudden activation, first lean into resourcing. What resource might you be able to lean into right now as you notice the activation arise? Can you co-regulate with a partner or safe friend (or imagine that they're there)? Can you orient to the space, allowing your eyes, ears, or nose to wander to something that's more pleasant to notice? Maybe you are wearing a special piece of jewelry, say a ring from your grandmother. Can you kinesthetically (through touch) orient to it, allowing yourself to feel its grooves, textures, and temperature? Choose something to focus on that will create a feeling of safety for you.
   » As you begin to notice your one resource, can you track what subtle shifts occur inside your body? Maybe you are able to breathe

more deeply, or you feel an easing in your muscles and facial expression. You might feel more present and grounded in your body and senses, experience pleasant emotions, or sense your body temperature coming back to neutral and your heartbeat slowing. As you notice these signs of deactivation and "counter-vortex," try to deepen and savor those sensations by slowing down and leaning into them.

2. **Pendulate:**

   » Now you can slowly pendulate your awareness back to the person whose presence is activating your nervous system. Perhaps you don't even have to look at them, but can just feel into their presence. As you do that, what might you begin to notice from your body?

   » Using interoception or SIBAM, you can track the experience of activation in your body—knowing that if it starts to feel like *too much, too soon, too fast*, you can dip right back out by pendulating to your resource, your anchor of safety. As you allow yourself to be in this somatic experience (the discomfort in your body) without judgment and without the desire to make it go away or to "fix the feeling," keep yourself open to what might happen next.

3. **Somatic completion:**

   » As you stay with the somatic experience and give it time (maybe you feel your heart beating faster, your palms sweating, your breath becoming shallow, a tightening in your body, etc.), does it initiate new impulses, desires, or experiences? Consider this as moving up the Polyvagal Ladder into mobilization, on the path to the ventral state at the top.

   » Perhaps you have the urge to look this person in the face boldly, or you have an impulse to allow yourself to turn and walk away or even just position yourself away from this person (rather than staying here in shutdown). You might want to clench your fists to feel your innate power. Or maybe you have a softer impulse to hold your partner's hand (sensing into the support that you have now and perhaps didn't have when the harm occurred).

4. **Discharge:**

   » In being with the experience of your body, and expressing what perhaps it wanted to happen all along, there likely will be a natural discharge felt in the form of trembling, tingling, heat, spontaneous deep breath, relaxed muscles, or expansion.

5. **Resource:**

   » Now as you pendulate back to your resource, can you anchor yourself back into your counter-vortex of regulation? Just like before, as you begin to notice your one resource, can you track what subtle shifts might occur inside? This healing vortex will likely feel even more expanded than before. This could be deeper breathing, easing in your muscles, a softer facial expression, feeling even more present and grounded in your body and senses, pleasant emotions, body temperature coming back to neutral, and a regular heartbeat. As you notice these signs of deactivation and counter-vortex, can you really deepen and savor those sensations by slowing down and leaning into them?

Somatic healing is about more than addressing trauma—it is a practice for rekindling your life energy (healthy stress hormones) that have been held hostage to a life of survival. The following chapters explain how to do the hands-on work to reconnect with the innate and primal wisdom of your body and set yourself free from the protective stronghold of your nervous system. When your life energy is released, it brings you back to joy, meaning, purpose, and vitality.

Glossary of Terms

Here's a glossary of terms along with a deeper explanation of each concept:

Capacity: The nervous system's resilience or ability to experience and contain feelings, both pleasant and unpleasant.

Discharge: A transitional response following a completed protective or defensive response. A natural discharge of survival hormones (adrenaline and cortisol) is usually experienced through heat, shaking, trembling, tingling, or other movements you can find on the lists on page 194 in this chapter.

Felt sense: A bodily awareness or intuition of your emotions, sensations, and experiences.

Healing/counter-vortex: In contrast to the trauma vortex, the healing/counter-vortex is our state of expansion and deactivation. Here, we are resourced and regulated. The counter-vortex represents our state of safety and connection (ventral vagal).

Interoception: A conscious internal awareness of the body.

Pendulation: The natural oscillating back and forth between states of contraction (trauma vortex) and expansion (counter-vortex) in the nervous system. Consider this your biorhythm.

Proprioception: The body's ability to sense itself in space and time.

Regulation: The body's ability to self-regulate and seek a natural balance and equilibrium between contraction (activation) and expansion (deactivation).

Resource: Anything internal or external that brings a felt sense of calm, safety, presence, grounding, or okayness.

SIBAM: The five elements of embodying an experience: Sensation, Image, Behavior, Affect, and Meaning.

Somatic completion/renegotiation: When our nervous system has the experience of "doing now what I couldn't do back then." This means that a protective or defensive response was finally initiated in the nervous system (to move away, to move toward, to protect or defend yourself or others, or to have time to orient to an oncoming threat), allowing the trauma to be renegotiated.

Titration: Moving at a slow and gentle pace.

Trauma vortex: The consumption of daily life by trauma that overwhelms our nervous system's capacity to cope. We either get sucked up in the vortex or are constantly running from it. The trauma vortex represents states of contraction and activation (fight, flight, shutdown).

CHAPTER 10

Self-Guided Experiencing: Before You Begin

The following six chapters will give you step-by-step instructions for self-guided somatic practices. Each will cover one of the Somatic Roadmaps as well as a Somatic Tools Library for the five stuck nervous system states (fight, flight, shutdown, functional freeze, and fawn). Chapter 16 provides guided *resourcing* practices for everyday situations and challenges. But first, I want to share some information that is crucial in making these experiences safe and gentle.

Somatic Experiencing Is a Way of Life

It is important to understand that healing your nervous system isn't a short-term commitment. Rather, it's a lifestyle change that starts slowly and gently and builds up over time. Remember that you are working with biological, automatic, and subconscious behaviors, beliefs, and emotions that were likely hardwired into your system long ago. So you should anticipate that building new neural networks and patterns—which promote new habitual responses—will take time. Change won't happen overnight, and it won't feel sudden; instead, it will feel gradual, subtle, almost nonexistent . . . until one day, you realize that life looks and feels different.

Think of it like going to the gym to build strength and resilience in your muscles. You start with lighter weights to avoid injuries. Then you increase the weight and intensity over time as your strength builds. You won't see the physical changes overnight, but if you stay committed to your workout routines and lifestyle, you may look back one day and realize that you look and feel like a completely different person.

This is what I want for you: a titrated healing process that provides more sustainability and promise for the long haul. You may want to rush the process and "just heal already." And believe me, I absolutely get it. You've struggled, suffered, and survived for a long time! You're exhausted, and you're just ready to be done living and feeling this way. But as much as you want to urgently get into the healing, what your body really *needs* is a pace that's slow—a pace that allows your system to be in the here and now, rather than being stuck in the turbulent trauma vortex of the past.

This slowing down is actually one of the biggest components of the healing.

And yet, this is where I see a lot of my clients get hung up—they don't think their healing is *fast enough* or *big enough*. This can lead to limiting beliefs like *I'm not doing enough, I'll never get better,* or *But I have to fix myself.* When this happens, I often will kindly remind them that we want to get them out of the chaos of *too much, too fast, too soon.* Further, the pressure we place on ourselves to heal creates further stress on the system. But because urgency might be what they are familiar with, it's what they subconsciously desire. I bring it back to the basics, that our aim isn't to make the discomfort go away, but rather to increase their resilience to be with that discomfort, thereby decreasing its impact over time.

Somatic Experiencing Tools Are Temporary

The tools and practices you will read about in the rest of the chapters in this book are meant to serve as a temporary support as you build organic somatic and nervous system resilience.

Let's revisit the analogy of the shallow hole in the sand. When your capacity to contain discomfort is too small, there may be times when a somatic tool can support you in decreasing or expelling the overwhelm. In the analogy of the sand hole, you can consider these somatic tools as small sand buckets that can aid you in emptying the water (the discomfort) that floods your shallow hole in the sand (your capacity). Although these tools can provide temporary relief from anything that feels like *too much*, *too soon*, *too fast*, you don't want to become completely dependent on these practices to move out of discomfort.

When we look to some of the emerging content surrounding somatic healing and nervous system regulation, there seems to be a glorification of the somatic tools and the quick fixes, without an equal focus on the fact that although they are useful, the end goal of nervous system healing is to create a greater capacity to be *in our body* rather than rushing to fix it, release it, or move through it. We don't want to have to rush to our sand bucket anytime water (or discomfort) enters the sand hole. We need to give the water time to be absorbed into the sand so it can erode and expand the hole, creating that deeper well of capacity. The goal is for you to become comfortable and consistent with the somatic process so that the nervous system will become adept at naturally pendulating back and forth on its own, without your prompting or intervening. Reflecting once more on the grandfather clock, the tools can help nudge the pendulum when it's stuck, with the ultimate purpose to bring that pendulum back into its own automatic rhythm between activation and deactivation.

At the end of the day, these tools will not heal you. This book will not heal you. Somatic Experiencing will not heal you. *You* heal you. The roadmap in this book simply leads you back to *yourself* and to the innate resources within you to *self-heal*. No one and nothing can heal you better than you can. You were built for it, designed for it; it's in your biology.

Some Gentle Healing Reminders

- In healing, small steps are big steps.

- As you heal, your body comes alive again, as if it is experiencing the world for the first time. Uncomfortable emotions or sensations are normal.

- It takes your body only ninety seconds to metabolize or move through an emotion, sensation, or feeling, even the difficult ones.

- When a body has been stuck in a survival state, it's sometimes harder to feel joy and safety than it is to feel discomfort. Growing a capacity to resource is just as important, if not more important, than growing a capacity for what doesn't feel good.

- Triggers are normally memories from the past or emotional age regressions. When they come up, release any judgment and tend to that younger part of you.

- Healing looks different for everyone.

- Trauma also looks different for everyone.

- In moments of self-judgment or criticism, present yourself with the Three C Inquiry: *curiosity, context,* and *compassion,* as you learned about on page 165.

- Healing isn't supposed to look pretty. Hard days are a part of the journey.

- Rest is necessary, productive, and doesn't need to be earned.

- This is a lifelong process. No need to rush it!

Somatic Roadmaps

Each of the roadmaps will provide a detailed example and walk-through of how you can use Somatic Experiencing to begin the process of *getting unstuck* from each of the five stuck personalities/states.

Realize that although these roadmaps are common approaches for these stuck states, not each example or suggestion illustrated will have the same effect on your unique nervous system. This chapter is meant to provide you with inspiration and a deeper preview of how to incorporate Somatic Experiencing into your healing.

A Review of the Five Steps of Somatic Experiencing

Before you explore these roadmaps, let's review the five steps of Somatic Experiencing:

1. **Resource:** Create a felt sense of safety (your supportive healing/counter-vortex).
2. **Pendulate:** Using titration, gently touch into the trauma vortex or discomfort by using interoception or SIBAM to notice how your body is experiencing this moment.
3. **Somatic completion:** Is there a *natural impulse* (don't force it!) to express or respond in a way you couldn't before?
4. **Discharge:** This will naturally follow completion. (You may feel tingling, shaking, or heat in your body, or cry, etc.)
5. **Resource:** Anchor back into your initial resource.

Somatic Tools Library

As mentioned at the beginning of this chapter, each Somatic Roadmap for the five stuck personalities/states will be followed by a Somatic Tools Library. Consider these tools to be the sand buckets you can use either when your system needs a resource or support or when your system has the capacity for a gentle nudge in the somatic completion phase. Below, you'll find a short introduction with instruction on *how* to use the tools, *when* to use the tools, and how you'll know they're working.

The somatic tools will help you either resource into your body or environment (down-regulate) when the activation feels like too much, or gently engage a mobilizing impulse to express or respond in a way you couldn't before (up-regulate).

Keep in mind that every nervous system is unique, so these tools will land differently for everyone. A few of these practices may not have an impact for you or might even have the opposite effect. This makes titration and pendulation especially important as you experiment. At the beginning, be sure to slowly dip into these practices so you can sense what supports you and what doesn't. When it feels like *too much*, you can pendulate back to your resources immediately. Don't forget that you also have agency to titrate a tool even more. If the physical action feels like *too much*, could you instead just imagine or visualize doing that action? For instance, instead of clenching your fists into a ball when you feel the impulse of fight, could you instead visualize clenching your fists and see what happens? Take your time so you can attune to what supports your system best.

The Basic Rules for Using the Somatic Tools

- **Keep it brief:** Only do these practices for a few minutes at most.

- **Start with one tool:** Using one tool at a time is best. For example, it's not suggested that you jump from one tool (like a few minutes of heel drops) to the next (like running in place for a few minutes). Doing too much can overwhelm your nervous system.

- **Use these tools when you are comfortable:** You can use these tools and practices anywhere you feel at ease, whether it's in your office, your bedroom, your car (although maybe not when you are driving), or a public space. As we saw in a previous chapter, you can even process your activation in a social gathering in a way that is subtle and discreet.

How to Know Your Somatic Experiencing Tools Are Working

Fortunately, there are many signs that the tools are working:

- Your body will have involuntary physical responses highlighting that either a new impulse is being initiated or a discharge is occurring. This can be yawning; swallowing; sighing; stretching; moving; changing posture; tingling in the fingers, arms, toes, or limbs; and/or coolness coming out through your limbs or even in your head.

- You might feel lighter in your body, coupled with a sense of relief, release, or an easing of tension.

- You feel yourself settling down. Your heart rate and breathing slow back to normal.

- Your body temperature regulates.

- You have more clarity in your mind and your thoughts.

- You feel more present in the space around you and feel more present in your body. For example, you may be able to feel the physical connection between your chair and your sit-bones.

- It's easier to be more open and receptive to connection with others.

It's helpful to track the intensity of what you're feeling either on a scale of one to ten, with ten being the most intense, or 1 to 100 percent, again, with 100 percent being the most intense. For instance, you might note that *The tension in my chest feels at about a seven* if using the one-to-ten scale. As you use the tools, notice any subtle or micro-changes to the scale; these don't need to be big. Even a one-point shift is a sign that it's working.

CHAPTER 11

Anger and the Armor of Fight

A nger is an essential and primary emotion, and one that we shouldn't be afraid of. We use anger to tap into our healthy aggression, what Peter Levine refers to as our *vitality* and *life force*. It's this innate power and aliveness that instills in us the sense of *I can do this, I am powerful, I am worthy*. Anger is the healing balm for suppression and shame, which live in the immobilizing states of shutdown, functional freeze, and fawn. We use our healthy aggression and life force to set and maintain boundaries, to defend ourselves or others, to advocate for ourselves, to speak our truth (therefore attracting deeper and healthier connections), and to propel us in life. Without anger on our side, we become stagnant, disconnected from ourselves, and ruled over by other people's agendas and desires.

Every holiday season I have an influx of clients in my practice who need support. Believe it or not, it's the most common season for anger to arise. Starting in November and carrying through the new year, there's always a buildup of activation and anticipation around attending the obligatory family gatherings and social events, where we know we'll be seeing the very people who trigger us—perhaps the people who harmed us, who belittled us, and who still attempt to keep us small even in our adult age. It's at these dysfunctional family events that we know our frustration will rise, only to be pushed back down because that's how it's always been, especially with *these people*. That's the mask, the armor we always wore—shutdown, suppress, appease, or avoid. When we were younger that likely made sense, because who knew what punishment or disconnection waited on the other side. And then there are those of us who are overflowing with anger we've never expressed, which seems to billow out every time we're around *these people*.

In this environment, where we often revert to the childlike parts of us (who either shut down, have a tantrum, run away, or appease), we might find ourselves triggered and activated by the seemingly smallest things. To those younger parts that armor up when we walk in that door, that smallest trigger can still feel like a matter of life and death.

I recall my client Kristi coming into a session full of rage, resentment, and shame following a Christmas dinner where her father had raised his voice at her young daughter for stealing an innocent bite of apple pie before it was served, disciplining her in the same demoralizing way he had always used with Kristi. Although Kristi wanted to defend her daughter, to step in and give her father a piece of her mind, she instead froze like a deer in the headlights. It was an automatic response, one that was all too familiar. It wasn't until she saw the heartbreak on her daughter's face that she was able to thaw out of her disbelief. It was in that moment that she excused the both of them, sneaking off to another room to allow her daughter's tears to flow in isolation—just like Kristi used to do. By the time she made it to our session, she was distraught with guilt. "I didn't protect her," she told me, "I'm so weak. I'm a horrible mother."

It was in that session that we began to gently tap into the innate healthy aggression and life force that had been thwarted in Kristi's life for far too long. She imagined herself as a mother bear—a powerful and competent protector. Oscillating between resource and activation, Kristi allowed the mobilizing fight energy to flow through her during the course of the session. It travelled to her limbs, radiating from her large muscle groups, propelling her after some time to stand tall and brave. She imagined herself as the powerful protector her daughter needed in that moment, and the one young Kristi had needed all along. It was a powerful experience, and an emotional one, as Kristi was able to finally rise in her power, allowing her to begin to restore the organic impulses that gave way to a sense of empowerment and confidence.

This example is for anger that arises during family gatherings, as described above.

1. **Resource:** In a situation like a family gathering, or any environment where *you know* you are very likely to be triggered into anger, it can be helpful to plan ahead by having a resource ready. For instance, if you know your partner or someone close to you is going to be there, you could perhaps ask them to be your co-regulator to lean on. I often use my husband in this way—he knows that if I spontaneously hold his hand that I'm looking for an anchor.

   If you don't have someone at the event for support, you could plan to use exploratory orienting (taking in the environment with your senses) or kinesthetic orienting (resourcing with an object through touch). I have clients who carry essential oils with them at all times, for instance, so they can orient to the soothing and calming smell to help them ground back into the present; others like to wear a piece of jewelry or simply orient to the texture of their clothes. You want your resource to be something to help you get in touch with the present moment. As you resource and begin to build your counter-vortex, you'll take an internal/interoceptive inventory of how that resource lands in your body—for instance, a settling, deeper breath or more awareness of the present moment, etc. You can deepen the resource by using the channels of SIBAM (Sensation, Image, Behavior, Affect, and Meaning) to track this experience.

2. **Pendulate:** Now, in the moments when anger presents itself, you want to start by gently dipping into that experience in the body—the trauma vortex or activation. Titration here is key. For now, you are simply observing and experiencing, not expressing or expelling. Questions you could ask would be *How am I noticing this anger? How is my body showing me I am angry?* You are tracking the interoceptive experience (sensation, feeling, emotion) and noticing its intensity. The elements of SIBAM can be helpful as well (see page 193). Pendulate back and forth from activation to resource if the activation starts to feel like *too much*.

3. **Somatic:** Completion As you're allowing your body to tolerably be in the trauma vortex of anger, look for any shifts or impulses that your body wants to do something, like express, move, or act. If an organic response emerges, slowly allow that completion to occur (like simply allowing the heat to rise and not pushing it away, clenching your fists, standing up, giving a defensive and empowered gaze, puffing up your chest, setting a boundary, saying no, etc.). Always titrate your response.

   If your system needs a gentle nudge and has the capacity for it, reference the Somatic Tools Library for Anger at the end of this chapter.

4. **Discharge:** As you are now being with the experience of your body and expressing what perhaps you wanted to happen all along, there likely will be a natural discharge of survival hormones. This will be felt in the form of trembling, tingling, heat, spontaneous deep breaths, relaxed muscles, or expansion. Allow this discharge to naturally occur, which will bring you back into deactivation.

5. **Resource:** Pendulating back to your resource, can you anchor yourself back into your counter-vortex of regulation? Just like before, as you begin to notice your one resource, can you track

what subtle shifts might occur inside? This could include deeper breathing, easing in your muscles, a softer facial expression, feeling more present and grounded in your body and senses, pleasant emotions, body temperature coming back to neutral, a regular heartbeat. As you notice these signs of regulation and counter-vortex, can you really deepen and savor those sensations by slowing down and leaning into them? Finally, to bring yourself into a moment of integration, does this experience now carry a different meaning? For instance, *I am powerful, I am deserving, I am capable, and I am safe.* As you notice this new and emerging story, try to notice what that's like in your body to be with that meaning.

Somatic Tools Library for Anger and the Armor of Fight

The goal: To engage overall mobilization in your body, specifically the defensive impulses of power, healthy aggression, and life force energy that have been thwarted. Use these tools in step 3, somatic completion, when your system has capacity for a gentle nudge.

Exercises

- **Air scream:** Allow yourself to "silently scream."

- **Animal sounds:** Allow yourself to listen to recorded sounds of a wild and powerful animal (like a lion or bear). After one minute, track any shifts from your body. You can find these sounds online or via any streaming music service.

- **Clenched jaw rebound:** Allow the tension and clenching in your jaw to exist and then slowly allow your tongue to relax and your jaw to drop down and open.

- **Fist clench:** Clench your fists tightly.

- **Growl:** Allow out a long, low "Rarrrrrrrrr." To deepen the practice, add a pushing motion with your arms (either while you are sitting or standing).

- **Peripheral space boundary-setting:** Start by standing with your feet shoulder-width apart. Lightly bend your knees, putting your weight into your quadriceps muscles. Track how it feels to be grounded in your legs and feet while bringing awareness to your balance, stability, and center of gravity. Now, place your feet outside your shoulder width to move into a wider stance, allowing you to take up more space with your body. Again, put your weight into your quads and feet and track how this feels. If you'd like, feel free to shift your weight from right to left, allowing you to take up more space with your upper body. This exercise uses healthy aggression to set a boundary and take up space with your body. It strengthens your vestibular system (balance, stability, and center of gravity), which is in constant communication with your nervous system.

- **Pillow squeeze:** Slowly squeeze and tighten a pillow, first with your hands and then slowly adding in your arm muscles.

- **Posture rebound:** Using a pillow, desk, or table for support, release your head and neck and let your spine collapse. From this position, wait for an organic impulse to begin lifting and lengthening your spine upward, moving very slowly as if you were raising one vertebra at a time. Allow your neck and head to rise up last. Feel into your open chest and lifted chin at the end, and notice your power. This should be a slow process and take one or two minutes to complete. If it feels comfortable, you can add a Superman pose at the end.

- **Towel twist:** Twist a towel, blanket, or piece of cloth tightly as you feel the muscles in your hands and arms brace and tremble.

- **Wall pushes:** Face a wall and place your hands on the wall at about shoulder height. Move your feet back and attempt to push and walk through the wall using your full might. Do this for ten to twenty seconds and then take a ten- to twenty-second break. Repeat up to five times.

Visualizations

- **Competent protector:** Imagine that you have an ally; a protector; or a supportive person, animal, or archetype nearby who *has your back* in this moment. Imagine that they are right behind you, backing you up; or imagine them right next to you, ready to support.

- **"No"/"stop" visualization:** Imagine saying no or stop, imagine raising your hand to signal no or stop, allow yourself to say no or stop, and then allow your hand to slowly lift and extend to signal no or stop. Be sure to titrate this tool as it feels most comfortable for your system.

- **Protective animal:** Imagine yourself as a wild and powerful animal, puffed up and ready to defend (for example, a bear, lion, wolf, shark, dog, etc.).

- **Wise ancestor:** Visualize an ancestor in your family you sense holds wisdom and power. Now consider that the cells and genetic makeup of that person are also inherently a part of you. Your strength comes from their strength. As you consider this intergenerational wisdom and life force, what do you notice internally?

CHAPTER 12

Fear, Anxiety, and the Armor of Flight

A nxiety is a necessary and protective emotion rooted in fear—your flight response. It's part of the human condition, and it can be triggered by various everyday scenarios beginning from childhood, including stranger shyness, separation, weather events, darkness, nightmares, performance and school anxiety, germs, getting ill or harmed, peer rejection, and more. Fear is healthy and helpful, until that fear interferes with normal life. For some people, small changes or challenges can send them into a tailspin.

Anxiety, in its most basic definition, is a natural response to unfamiliar or overwhelming experiences. Remember, everything about you makes sense, including fear and anxiety. This is your body's alarm sending you a message, and ignoring the alarm doesn't make it go away. Attuning to the alarm by acknowledging and addressing it is what will support you.

This is why it can be frustrating to hear "Just calm down" when you're in the throes of anxiety. You might be trembling or shaking and attempting to will yourself to stop. Yet resisting the anxious alarm with *calm* is simply another form of avoidance (something those with a chronic flight response are good at, running away). It's as if we believe we're turning off the alarm, but we're really just pressing the snooze button—and it's always short-lived. Avoiding isn't the same thing as processing. The overwhelm of mobilizing survival hormones will still spill over at any minor stress.

Through a somatic lens, on the other hand, we recognize that your fear and anxiety have a purpose that hasn't been felt, and that, when given space and time to be slowly experienced, they will ultimately expel themselves naturally. In other words, that trembling and shaking is actually your body doing what it needs to do to discharge that excess stress.

One group in my practice that I commonly see affected by anxiety is new mothers. Women already have high levels of hormones during pregnancy, and those levels shift drastically after giving birth. Factor in the sleepless nights coupled with unrealistic expectations that first-time moms carry—well, who wouldn't be anxious! I remember how easy it was for my nervous system to perceive every sneeze or cough from my son as a danger signal after he was born. During the years, I've had numerous moms reach out to receive support for their anxiety, even after they've already had several children. For most of these mothers, I learned that the anxiety began after the first child but was pushed aside and ignored. Yet it persisted, keeping them stuck in chronic cycles of fear and worry.

ON TARGET!

My client Tess's first child had a serious medical scare as an infant. While the baby recovered, Tess's unresolved anxiety and worries after the birth of her second child became so overwhelming that she developed chronic health conditions that plagued her physical body, like early arthritis, and emotional symptoms like agoraphobia. She was unable to leave the house either alone or with her kids, for fear that they would get sick again. After working with her for a few months, I was thrilled to get this message:

> Britt, Holy cow. I did it. I went to Target all by myself last night. Even just a few months ago, it felt impossible. I thought my health was just so poor and that I would never be able to walk the Target (or any other store) aisles mindlessly by myself again. But I'm realizing that it was my anxiety holding me back. I literally hadn't been inside of a Target in over two years. I passed out while pregnant there once, and I thought being there would activate me, that I'd be thinking that it would happen again. It's crazy to see the past two years of my life through this new lens and see how being stuck in survival for so long created a ripple effect in all aspects of my life. I've been so emotional, so full of gratitude, and I'm so incredibly proud of myself for doing it, even when it felt hard. I'm slowly taking off the straitjacket that I have felt a prisoner to, and I'm feeling so full of hope.

This example is for nervous fliers. You can use these steps for any other anxious situation.

1. **Resource:** Before takeoff, or perhaps even before going to the airport, you should consider what's something that will help you feel safe and *resourced* during the flight. If you're flying with someone else, you could practice co-regulation by perhaps holding their hand or sharing your feelings, offering a chance for your system to be compassionately seen, heard, and held. If you're flying on your own, maybe there's an object, a picture on your phone, or a playlist that brings you comfort and could support you. If you don't have an object, perhaps you can feel the seat supporting your back, or focus on the face of the adorable baby in the seat across from you. As you resource and begin

to build your counter-vortex, track in your body how that *feels* pleasant to notice. Is there more ease in your shoulders, deeper breath, a loosening of your jaw, or a feeling more settled in the weight of your seat? Slowly track the interoceptive cues or channels of SIBAM.

2. **Pendulate:** Slowly shift your attention to the discomfort of the anxiety. Notice how your body is showing you it's anxious. Are you sweating? Is it difficult to breathe? Are you wringing your hands? Is there bracing or constriction in your chest? Get curious and observant about the activation that's happening in your body and nervous system as you dip into the trauma vortex—not pushing it away, but just being *with* it. Give the sensation an intensity rating, on a scale of one to ten, with ten being most intense. For instance, *The tightness in my throat is at about a seven right now.* Realize that you are tracking the interoceptive experience (sensation, feeling, emotion) and noticing its intensity. The elements of SIBAM can be helpful as well. Pendulate back and forth from activation to resource if the activation starts to feel like *too much.*

3. **Somatic completion:** You may find that just by taking time to notice the activation, it begins to decrease in intensity, followed by a natural discharge. If not, and you need gentle support to discharge, here's a possible tool to use: If you begin to notice a shift into impulse or expression, ask yourself, *What does my body want to do now?* As someone who travels a lot and sometimes gets anxious in stimulating environments, here are a few tools I've used to discharge the high-energy activation of anxiety and the flight response:

   First, I'll lightly shake out my limbs to engage the protective response to flee. I shake out my right hand for ten to fifteen seconds, followed by my right arm, my left hand, and then my left arm. When our body begins to involuntarily tremble, we don't want to push it away but instead give into the response. This is your body and physiology trying to naturally discharge and complete the stress response cycle.

Another tool I've used in this scenario is heel drops (think calf-raises). With one foot at a time, and alternating back and forth, I raise up on my toes, really engaging the muscles in my calf, and then drop my heel down to the ground. This movement mirrors the instinctive flight response to run away.

Lastly, I've utilized the armrest as an object to squeeze while feeling my muscles brace through my fingers, hands, and up into my arms. After thirty seconds of contraction, I release as expansion takes over. (This is similar to a pandiculation tool.)

If your system needs a gentle nudge and has the capacity for it, reference the Somatic Tools Library for Anxiety at the end of this chapter.

4. **Discharge:** When you stay with the experience of your body, there will likely be a natural discharge of survival hormones. You may experience trembling, tingling, heat, spontaneous deep breaths, relaxed muscles, or expansion. Allow this discharge to naturally occur, which will bring you back into deactivation.

5. **Resource:** Now, pendulate back to your resource and try to anchor yourself back into your counter-vortex of regulation. Just like before, as you begin to notice your resource try tracking what subtle shifts might occur inside. You may experience deeper breathing, easing in your muscles, a softer facial expression, feeling more present and grounded in your body and senses, or pleasant emotions. Your body temperature may return to neutral and you may have a more regular heartbeat. As you notice these signs of regulation and counter-vortex, try to deepen and savor those sensations by slowing down and leaning into them. Finally, bring yourself into a moment of integration. Consider: Does this experience now carry a different meaning?

For instance, you may think: *I am powerful, I am deserving, I am capable, I am safe.* As you notice this new and emerging story, try to notice what it feels like in your body to be with that meaning.

Somatic Tools Library for Anxiety and the Armor of Flight

The goal: To engage overall mobilization in our body, specifically the protective impulses of escape, power, and life force energy. Use these tools in step 3, somatic completion, when your system has capacity for a gentle nudge.

Exercises

- **Energy release:** Imagine first that you are standing and lifting a heavy boulder above your head and then slamming it down to the ground as the energy of adrenaline and cortisol release below you. If you're able to physically do this, stand with your feet apart, lift your hands above your head, and, as you brace your muscles, pull your hands and your body down as if you're throwing that imaginary boulder down to the ground below you. (It should almost look like you're skiing.) Do this with force. Repeat for up to one minute.

- **Free movement:** When you have mobilizing flight energy, you often feel antsy, fidgety, and restless. Tune into the potential movement that your body wants to participate in, and dance, stretch, play, roll, wrestle, run, etc.

- **Heel drops:** Lift onto your toes and forcefully allow your heels to drop into the ground, feeling the thud below. This is a quicker movement. Do this for up to one minute, dropping your heels once every second.

- **Heel pushes:** As you sit, push your heels down into the ground as if trying to break through the floor below you. Start with one foot at a time, noticing the bracing of your muscles through your foot, calf muscles, quadriceps, and glutes. Do this for up to one minute for each foot.

- **Heels up:** As you sit, lean forward in your seat while lifting your heels up and activating or engaging your calf muscles (as if you're about to get up and get away). Do this for one minute. If you feel that you have the capacity, you can deepen this practice by adding in three short and consecutive inhales at the end, further mobilizing your heart rate.

- **Labored breathing:** Allow for short and quick inhales and exhales for up to one minute.

- **Limb shaking:** Start by shaking one hand at a time, as if you're trying to shake water off your hands, then add one whole arm at a time. You also can shake out one foot at a time, followed by one whole leg at a time.

- **Pandiculation tense-and-relax sequence:** Pandiculation (an impulsive stretch) is your nervous system's brilliant way of waking up your sensorimotor system to prepare you to move or mobilize. This naturally happens when you yawn or wake up as a way to engage your arousal. Allow for a full-body stretch from head to toe—arms, fingers, palms, legs, toes, etc.—followed by releasing into relaxation and expansion.

- **Physiological sigh:** Allow for an inhale, but before you get to the top, take another inhale. Then, expel all your air with an exhale. (Feel free to add a vocal sigh to the exhale to activate the calming effects of the vagus nerve.) Do this for up to one minute.

- **Posture orienting:** Take notice of the nearest exit—that is, your *escape*. First, allow your eyes to orient to the exit, taking in the visual space for a minute. Next, if possible, position or posture your body to face the exit.

- **Posture rebound:** See page 226.

- **Run stance:** Assume a running posture or stance. Even while sitting, you can lean forward in a chair and position your feet so they're ready to propel you forward.

- **Running in place:** Run in place for up to one minute.

Visualizations

- **Breaking roots:** Visualize that your feet have roots in the ground, making it difficult to move or escape. Next, visualize that the roots are being broken away as your feet become free to move and mobilize.

- **Powerful animal:** Imagine yourself as a fast and powerful animal, ready to run away or escape.

CHAPTER 13

Depression, Burnout, and the Armor of Shutdown

Your dorsal vagal shutdown state is home to both depression and burnout. Here, we retreat into nothingness; numbness; and disconnection from self, from others, and from the world. Our biology has entered into a state of conservation and hibernation as all of our working systems have decelerated to the slowest possible speed, leaving only fumes to run on. Exhaustion and dissociation take over as a means to keep us still, ensuring conservation of energy. In recognizing that this is the bottom of the nervous system ladder, titration is especially important for the journey back up to the top, where safety and connection reside.

I want to reiterate that the state of shutdown has tremendous purpose. It's often necessary when the weight of life has become overwhelming. Often, I have clients who place judgment or criticism on themselves for being in this state, and in a world that glorifies mobilizing productivity, hustle culture, and the go-go-go lifestyle, I can see where those limiting beliefs can stem from. But I want to remind you of one thing: *rest is productive*. Rest allows for repair and then reorganizing for the climb back up the ladder. And the pace at which you climb that ladder is incredibly important. For instance, with chronic fatigue, in moments when you feel good or energized, it's crucial to save some of that energy and not spend it all. When coming out of shutdown, go slowly as you resume life-affirming activities; otherwise, you'll just continue the patterns that exhaust you. It's a marathon, not a sprint.

Luis was sixty-eight years old when he came to work with me and had been suffering from depression, isolation, and chronic fatigue for a number of years. He had been in and out of therapy for decades, and concluded that his symptoms could be attributed to a horrific heartbreak in his thirties and a traumatic financial loss in his forties. From our first session together, I could sense that he had spent most of his life in his head—analyzing and conceptualizing yet completely detached from feeling, which given his past trauma, made a lot of sense. Talking and thinking can be a management strategy to avoid or disconnect from difficult feeling.

Luis was as smart as they came and had read more traumatology books than any client I'd had previously. He likely knew more about the science of Somatic Experiencing than I did at the time. His mind was his escape, from what we'd later discover was a childhood void of the secure attachment he never knew he needed, a childhood with an absent father and a mother who never once said "I love you." He knew he was loved in theory, but he never *felt it* or was shown it physically. This absence of bonding created enormous fear—"terror" he'd call it—around connecting with others. He carried this highly charged and anxious terror as an excruciating and unbearably painful knot in his stomach. He said the knot pulled in two directions—one side desperately longing for connection and the other paralyzed by fear of connection. This pain would surface anytime we'd begin to move out of his normal dissociation and into feeling.

As the pieces of the puzzle began to come together, I helped Luis understand that his exhaustion was a direct mirror of how much terror he had, because that was the amount of energy needed to push down, suppress, or dissociate from the terror. No wonder he was so shut down and depleted. His system had been working so hard, for so long. When I shared this reflection, Luis wanted to dive into the terror so he could "get rid of the pain" or symptom, but I had to explain that we first needed to work with the dissociation, because somatic completion and renegotiation of that fear and terror weren't possible if we couldn't be present in the body.

Developmental trauma, like attachment trauma, always requires time and compassionate attention. Throughout our earlier sessions, Luis and I spent much of our time building a safe relational container, one where his system could first feel seen, held, and supported by mine. As we created a space of healthy co-regulation and began to build his capacity to be in his body, the next phase of our process naturally unfolded. During our time together, Luis's system began to thaw out, allowing for emotional imprints previously buried to emerge. This granted us opportunities to witness and tend to those younger parts of Luis, allowing the feelings of the past to be experienced, expressed, and renegotiated in an empowering and beautiful way.

The example below will walk you through the earlier stages of first building capacity to be in the body from a place of shutdown.

This example is for anyone who is feeling shut down, depressed, burnt out, or exhausted.

1. **Resource:** In a state of shutdown, you want to resource with something that is going to bring you either into your body or your environment, keeping you grounded in the present. Resources that can bring you into presence could include kinesthetic orienting (through touch) or exploratory orienting (through the senses). As you resource and begin to build your counter-vortex, track in your body how that *feels* pleasant to notice. Is there more ease in your shoulders, are your breaths deeper, is your jaw looser, and are you feeling more settled in the

weight of your seat? Slowly track the interoceptive cues or channels of SIBAM.

2. **Pendulate:** From here, slowly shift your awareness to the discomfort you notice in your body, remembering to really titrate this step because your system needs a lot of space and time to process from a state of shutdown. If dissociation occurs, either from the body or from the mind, it's important to track what keeps you present, as you also track the *leaving feeling* of dissociation. (This is explained in more detail in the next section on functional freeze.) You might be wondering how you track dissociation when you feel nothing. Remember that "numb" and "spacey" are still feelings. If possible, can you track what qualities it has? Is it dark, hazy, or foggy in your mind? Does the numbness cover just your feet, your legs, or your lower body? Do they feel heavy, frozen, or floaty? Remember that dissociation is simply a natural response to something that feels overwhelming. It has good intentions and doesn't have to be feared. Again, you are tracking the interoceptive experience (sensation, feeling, emotion) and noticing their intensity. The elements of SIBAM can be helpful as well. Pendulate back and forth from activation to resource if the activation starts to feel like *too much*.

3. **Somatic completion:** As you gently and tolerably experience the trauma vortex of shutdown, look for any shifts or impulses that your body wants to do something, like express, move, or act. If an organic response emerges, slowly allow that completion to occur. Remember to titrate your response. Natural responses could look like allowing tears to flow, giving into the impulse to stretch, wanting to change your environment, or feeling a rise in the spine.

    If your system needs a gentle nudge and has the capacity for it, reference the Somatic Tools Library for Shutdown at the end of this chapter.

4. **Discharge:** As you are now being with the experience of your body and expressing what perhaps you wanted to happen all along, there likely will be a natural discharge of survival hormones. You may feel this in the form of trembling, tingling, heat, spontaneous deep breaths, relaxed muscles, or expansion. Allow this discharge to naturally occur, which will bring you back into deactivation.

5. **Resource:** Now, pendulate back to your resource and try to anchor yourself back into your counter-vortex of regulation. Just like before, as you begin to notice your resource, try tracking what subtle shifts might occur inside. You may experience deeper breathing, easing in your muscles, a softer facial expression, feeling more present and grounded in your body and senses, or pleasant emotions. Your body temperature may return to neutral and you may have a more regular heartbeat. As you notice these signs of regulation and counter-vortex, try to deepen and savor those sensations by slowing down and leaning into them. Finally, bring yourself into a moment of integration. Consider: Does this experience now carry a different meaning? For instance, you may think: *I am powerful, I am deserving, I am capable, I am safe.* As you notice this new and emerging story, try to notice what it feels like in your body to be with that meaning.

Somatic Tools Library for Depression, Burnout, and the Armor of Shutdown

The goal: To get back into our bodies and back into the present moment. To allow rest and to lightly engage mobilization to begin to move up the nervous system ladder. Use these tools in either step 2, pendulation, when your system needs more presence or resource, or step 3, somatic completion, when your system has capacity for a gentle nudge.

Exercises

- **Acupuncture mat:** Use an acupuncture mat to engage tactile (touch) and proprioceptive (muscle and joint) awareness. Touch brings you back into your body, as does the pressure you apply with your muscles into the mat (proprioception).

- **Auricular nerve (ear) massage:** The vagus nerve connects to the auricular nerves in your ears. This is why we "perk up" when we're on edge. Massaging your ears stimulates the auricular nerves and, therefore, the vagus nerve. Gently pull your ears away from your head. Lightly pull them back and hold. Lightly pull them outward and hold. Lightly pull them up and hold. Lastly, lightly pull them down and hold. Next, use your index finger to gently massage directly behind the lower part of the ear, in front of the ear, and in the concha (the hollow area right outside of the ear canal).

- **Butterfly hug:** This is a form of bilateral stimulation. Cross your arms over your chest while gently and slowly tapping your shoulders, alternating from left to right rhythmically with your hands.

- **Containment:** Consider that your body is your container. Begin to slowly pat your body all over, taking time to notice where your *edges* are. Sense into the feeling of having edges. This is the place where you end and the rest of the world begins.

- **"Easier to be with":** In moments when you notice parts of your body that are either in pain or dissociated, ask yourself, *Is there a part of my body in this moment that's easier to be with?* It could be your feet, your fingers, your neck, etc. Then, bring your interoceptive (sensations) or proprioceptive (muscles, joints) awareness to that place.

- **Head cradle:** Place your right hand on your forehead and your left hand on the back of your neck at the base of your head (occipital bone). Apply gentle pressure to these areas, allowing for deep breaths.

- **Heel pushes:** See page 234.

- **Muscle massage:** To wake up your proprioceptive system (which senses into your muscles, joints, and skin and communicates with the nervous system), give yourself a gentle muscle massage.

- **Peripheral gaze:** Your gaze shifts from state to state based on how your nervous system is orienting to the space around you. When you are in defensive orienting, your pupils dilate and your gaze becomes narrow, scanning for threats. When you are in exploratory orienting, your pupils are wide and your gaze becomes peripheral, allowing you to take in more of the world around you. Allow both of your hands to point with just your index finger. Next, raise your arms straight out in front of you at shoulder height, and bring your hands and index fingers side by side, touching each other in a parallel fashion. With your fingers pointed upward, allow your eyes to fixate on your fingers for up to one minute, taking in the details. Now, without moving your eyes, start to slowly separate your arms and fingers, still raised at shoulder height, pulling them slowly out to your sides and stopping at the edge of your peripheral gaze. (You should still be able to see them out of the corner of your eye without directly looking.) Lower your hands and allow yourself to explore and orient to the space around you with this wide peripheral gaze.

- **Rocking and swaying:** This is a form of bilateral stimulation and a procedural pattern of self-soothing from infancy. Allow yourself to gently rock or sway from side to side.

- **Somatic Experiencing self-hug:** Place your right hand just below your left armpit as you hold the side of your chest, feeling your heartbeat beneath your palm. Place your left hand on your right shoulder or arm, allowing yourself a gentle holding or hug. Be with this exercise for a minute or two, allowing yourself to breathe into your body and heart.

- **VOO:** Take in a deep breath. As you exhale, make a low and long "VOOOO" sound, drawing out the last vowel (so you sound like a foghorn). You will feel this low sound reverberate through your chest and even down to your belly. Repeat for up to one minute.

Visualization

- **SIFT:** This acronym stands for "sensation, image, feeling, thought." You'll spend up to one minute with each category. First, bring to mind a memory that felt pleasant, or imagine a moment that could feel pleasant. As you observe this memory or moment, you're going to identify, in order (1) the sensations you experienced in that memory—temperature, sound, smell, taste, etc.; (2) the image of what you see, taking in all the details—textures, objects, colors, patterns, people, faces, etc.; (3) the feelings you experienced in your body, which can be emotions or an internal felt sense—joy, openness, love, expanded, peace, relaxed, etc.; and (4) the thoughts or stories you're telling yourself in that moment or memory—*Life is beautiful, I'm safe in this moment,* etc.

CHAPTER 14

Dissociation and the Armor of Functional Freeze

As mentioned in the previous chapter, dissociation is a *feeling*, even though the feeling is one of numbness or nothingness. Functional freeze, which is a blended state of shutdown and flight, can be characterized as the state of autopilot. In this state, we have mobilizing energy to *go through the motions*, yet our shutdown state pulls us down into the *suppression of our emotions*. Just as the name implies, we're functioning and going about our daily lives, yet we feel little to nothing.

Many parents, especially those who stay at home with their young children while their partner works out of the house, can feel trapped by the endless chores, the needs of their little ones, the lack of sleep and ensuing extreme fatigue, the housekeeping duties, the errands, and more. They can't quit by running away or shutting down, because they have to tend to the children who depend on them. They're stuck between a rock and hard place, likely thinking: *"I want to take a break, but I can't."* This is the reality of functional freeze, when we're here but not really present.

Julie was a single mom who was overwhelmed by the constant stress of motherhood. With three school-age children, her time was consumed with scheduling all their events, drop-offs and pickups, and making the meals, all while working part-time to alleviate her precarious financial situation. Life was understandably a lot. It made sense when Julie would show up to our sessions dissociated, sharing through an emotionless expression that things were "just fine" and that she was also doing "just fine"—when both of us knew she wasn't. On the outside, she appeared calm under pressure; on the inside, she was in utter turmoil. In the same way that I first worked with Luis's shutdown response before moving into his fear, functional freeze follows the same path and approach. In recognizing that part of Julie needed to thaw out first, we took time in our sessions to focus on her shutdown and dissociation response before moving to her mobilizing response. As always when working with blended states, we start with the slowest part of you.

This example is for anyone who is in overwhelm from parenting or from any stressful situation that doesn't seem to have an end in sight.

1. **Resource:** For dissociation, it helps to resource with something that is going to bring you back to the present, either in your body or in your environment. A question to ask yourself could be, *How do I know I'm here right now?* You can notice how firmly you are sitting in a chair, or how your feet are flat on the ground, or how your chest is moving up and down with every breath. Or you can bring your attention to your senses; focus on something pleasant that you can see, touch, hear, smell, or taste. As you resource and begin to build your counter-vortex, track in your body how that *feels* pleasant to notice. Is there more ease in your shoulders, are you taking deeper breaths, does your jaw feel looser, do you feel more settled in the weight of your seat? Slowly track the interoceptive cues or channels of SIBAM.

2. **Pendulate:** When you start to pendulate, you're going to dip one toe into the dissociation yet keep the other foot in the present. For example, ask yourself if there is a place that feels more present in your body. Maybe it's your back against the chair, for instance. As you notice that support on your back, can you also at the same time notice the place that feels dissociated or numb? And then from this place of being anchored in another area of the body, can you begin to track that numbness? How might you feel that numbness? How might you describe it? What I often hear is that it feels foggy, empty, or heavy; it looks like the image of a floating balloon; or it has a color to it (usually white).

Again, you are tracking the interoceptive experience (sensation, feeling, emotion) and noticing their intensity. The elements of SIBAM can be helpful as well. Pendulate back and forth from activation to resource if the activation starts to feel like *too much*.

3. **Somatic completion:** From the trauma vortex of dissociation, some things to get curious about are *How can I come back into my body and bring more presence there?* and *How can I encourage a little bit of mobilization or natural impulse?* Perhaps you could start by just *imagining* that you are moving your limbs. If your feet are numb, can you imagine moving your right foot without actually moving it? Or could you imagine that your foot is pushing up and down on a gas pedal? And as you imagine that, what happens next? Is there a natural impulse now to either apply pressure, move slightly, shift, or brace that part of your body? This time, allow yourself to very slowly move your foot up and down as if you really are in a car.

When working with dissociation, this step of the process needs to be much more titrated than in the other four states in this chapter. You want to integrate these steps even more slowly than you think you need to. Imagine or visualize first, and then actually make the movement.

If your system needs a gentle nudge and has the capacity for it, reference the Somatic Tools Library for Functional Freeze at the end of this chapter.

4. **Discharge:** As you are now being with the experience of your body, and expressing what perhaps you wanted to happen all along, there likely will be a natural discharge of survival hormones. This will be felt in the form of trembling, tingling, heat, spontaneous deep breaths, relaxed muscles, or expansion. Allow this discharge to naturally occur, which will bring you back into deactivation.

5. **Resource:** Now, pendulate back to your resource and try to anchor yourself back into your counter-vortex of regulation. Just like before: as you begin to notice your resource, try tracking what subtle shifts might occur inside. You may experience deeper breathing, easing in your muscles, a softer facial expression, feeling more present and grounded in your body and senses, or pleasant emotions. Your body temperature may return to neutral and you may have a more regular heartbeat. As you notice these signs of regulation and counter-vortex, try to deepen and savor those sensations by slowing down and leaning into them. Finally, bring yourself into a moment of integration. Consider: Does this experience now carry a different meaning? For instance, you may think: *I am powerful, I am deserving, I am capable, I am safe.* As you notice this new and emerging story, try to notice what it feels like in your body to be with that meaning.

Somatic Tools Library for Dissociation and the Armor of Functional Freeze

The goal: To get back into your body and back to the present moment. To rest and to lightly engage in mobilization to begin to move up the nervous system ladder. Use these tools in either step 2, pendulation, when your system needs more presence or resource, or step 3, somatic completion, when your system has capacity for a gentle nudge.

Exercises

- **Auricular nerve (ear) massage:** See page 241.

- **Body scan for numbness:** Remember that numbness is a feeling; you *feel* numb, therefore you can track it and explore its boundaries. First, begin by asking yourself: "Is it ok to notice that there's numbness here?" Begin to track where you feel this numbness. Now, in exploring its boundaries, you can map the edges where the sensation of numbness meets the sensation of presence within your body. How is it to notice that boundary, to recognize that not all of you is numb? Can you imagine different colors for these two different sensations? And as you bring awareness to these different sensations, can you imagine the presence flowing into the numbness?

- **Chair drops:** This tool strengthens your vestibular system (balance, stability, and center of gravity), which is in constant communication with your nervous system. While sitting down on a chair, gently lift the front of the chair up and backward (either with your feet or hands) allowing the front legs of the chair to rise above the ground up to six inches. Don't lean back to the point of feeling like you don't have stability. Next, allow the front of the chair to drop back down—feeling the gravity of your body meet the ground, feeling the thud below. Do this slowly up to five times. As you do so, do you feel more weight in your body? Do you feel heavier? More grounded? More stable?

- **Co-regulation:** Spend time in connection with another living human or animal.

- **Free movement:** See page 233.

- **Heated hands:** Rub your hands together until you have created enough friction to create heat in your hands. When your hands are warm, allow both hands to lightly squeeze and massage your limbs. This is a form of temperature exposure.

- **Limb shaking:** See page 234.

- **Mindfulness sensory exercise:** This is a five-four-three-two-one exercise. Bring your conscious awareness to five things you can see, four things you can touch, three things you can hear, two things you can smell, and one thing you can taste.

- **New environment:** With the intention of reconnecting to your present environment, take yourself to a new environment, like going outside or into a new room.

- **Posture rebound:** See page 226.

- **Temperature change:** You can use warm or cold exposure to bring yourself back into the presence of your body. Options include standing in front of an open refrigerator or freezer for a minute or two, running cold water over your hands or splashing it on your face, holding frozen food, placing a cold washcloth on your face (which stimulates the vagus nerve), stepping outside where the temperature is different, feeling the sun on your skin, using a heated blanket, using a heating pad, or holding a warm cup of tea or coffee. (I do not recommend cold plunges or extended cold showers for those who have a dysregulated nervous system. Cold plunges are intended to be used to increase mental awareness and productivity, which happens through elevating your stress hormones. However, this shock can feel like *too much* for an overwhelmed nervous system that's already flooded with stress hormones, therefore potentially sending your system deeper into shutdown.)

- **Vestibular weight:** Your nervous system is always communicating with your vestibular system, which oversees your center of gravity and how your body holds your weight in space and time (your balance, weight, and stability). Start by standing with your feet shoulder-width apart. Give your legs a slight bend at the knees, and tuck your pelvic bone forward as you balance your weight across the full bed of your feet by standing on your toes and heels, not just leaning on your heels or on your toes. Stand here for a minute and then start to notice if you feel like your center of gravity is pulled forward, backward, to the left, or to the right. (These are the quadrants of your peri-personal space.) Now, without moving your feet, begin to shift your weight toward each quadrant, noticing how that feels to be in your body, in your weight, and in your center of gravity.

- **VOO:** See page 243.

Visualization

- **Thawing visualization:** Imagine a thawing-out process over any areas you feel are *frozen* or *numb*. Here's an example: imagine warm water running over your feet, which feel numb or dissociated, and visualize a thawing out, toe by toe, and working your way up. You can use whatever thawing imagery comes to mind (in front of a fire, a heat lamp, a hair dryer, etc.).

CHAPTER 15

Appeasement and the Armor of Fawn

F awn is a blended state of shutdown and flight. In this state, we have mobilizing energy to flee, run away, and avoid out of fear (usually of rejection or harm) and also have the immobilizing impulse to shut down and suppress our healthy aggression and vitality, our truth, our boundaries, and our authenticity in order to fit in.

Fawn often shows up in the workplace, where an inherent power dynamic already exists. Perhaps you don't want to upset your boss or ruffle feathers with your colleagues. This can lead to you saying yes to every single task that's asked of you, being overly agreeable, not asking for a raise when one is overdue, avoiding conflict or setting boundaries, and more. I've heard every one of these examples and more from my clients—and, of course, they have the added anxiety of worrying that they might be fired or demoted if they step into their power and healthy aggression.

This example is for anyone who feels the need to continually appease a person or people, either at work or in another setting.

1. **Resource:** It is helpful to keep something at your desk at work that you can easily pull out and orient to (like how I have my rocks from Glacier National Park in the pencil holder on my desk). This can be any kind of object that makes you feel grounded

or resourced, like something your child made for you, a small photo, or a candle. Or, if you're called into a meeting and don't have an object to touch, orienting can be helpful. Look around the room and fix your gaze on something that's pleasant or neutral to notice. As you resource and begin to build your counter-vortex, take an internal/interoceptive inventory of how that resource lands in your body—for instance, settling, deeper breaths, more awareness of the present moment, etc. You can deepen the resource by using the channels of SIBAM to track this experience.

2. **Pendulate:** As you pendulate into discomfort and the trauma vortex, what might you notice about the experience of your body? The most common emotions that arise in a fawning scenario are fear (which makes us avoid or shut down), coupled with anger that's suppressed (the healthy aggression we need to say or do what we really want to). Remember here that the fear is stopping you from being in your power and healthy aggression, so it has to be teased out and processed first. You want to be tracking the interoceptive experience (sensation, feeling, emotion) and noticing its intensity. The elements of SIBAM can be helpful as well. Pendulate back and forth from activation to resource if the activation starts to feel like *too much*.

3. **Somatic completion:** As you're allowing your body to tolerably be in the trauma vortex, look for any shifts or impulses that your body wants to do something, such as express, move, or act. If an organic response emerges, slowly allow that completion to occur, like simply allowing the heat to rise and not pushing it away, clenching your fists, standing up, giving a defensive and empowered gaze, puffing up your chest, setting a boundary, saying no, etc. Remember to titrate your response.

  If your system needs a gentle nudge and has the capacity for it, reference the Somatic Tools Library for Fawn at the end of this chapter.

4. **Discharge:** As you are now being with the experience of your body, and expressing what perhaps you wanted to happen all along, there likely will be a natural discharge of survival hormones. This will be felt in the form of trembling, tingling, heat, spontaneous deep breaths, relaxed muscles, or expansion. Allow this discharge to naturally occur, which will bring you back into deactivation.

5. **Resource:** Now, pendulate back to your resource and try to anchor yourself back into your counter-vortex of regulation. Just like before: as you begin to notice your resource, try tracking what subtle shifts might occur inside. You may experience deeper breathing, easing in your muscles, a softer facial expression, feeling more present and grounded in your body and senses, or pleasant emotions. Your body temperature may return to neutral and you may have a more regular heartbeat. As you notice these signs of regulation and counter-vortex, try to deepen and savor those sensations by slowing down and leaning into them. Finally, bring yourself into a moment of integration. Consider: Does this experience now carry a different meaning? For instance, you may think: *I am powerful, I am deserving, I am capable, I am safe.* As you notice this new and emerging story, try to notice what it feels like in your body to be with that meaning.

Somatic Tools Library for Appeasement and the Armor of Fawn

The goal: To engage overall mobilization in your body, specifically the defensive impulses of power, healthy aggression, and life force energy that have been thwarted.

The antidote to fawning is a healthy fight response. We set boundaries, advocate for ourselves, and rise into our power. Therefore, these tools mirror those for anger and the armor of fight in chapter 12. See page 225.

CHAPTER 16

Resourcing for Common Health Issues and Everyday Triggers

This chapter contains a list of common health issues, as well as activating experiences that can occur in your daily life, and describes how resourcing and the five steps of Somatic Experiencing can help. Keep in mind that every nervous system is unique, so these are simply suggestions to gently practice and see if they work for you.

As you know, trauma happens fast and healing happens slow, but the more you use these tools over time, slowly, the more these simple routines and techniques will create greater resilience in your nervous system. Remember that as you resource and begin to build your counter-vortex, take an internal/interoceptive inventory of how that resource lands in your body. For instance, do you feel a settling, a deeper breath, more awareness of the present moment, etc.? You can deepen the resource by using the channels of SIBAM to track this experience.

Attention Deficit Hyperactivity Disorder (ADHD)

To address ADHD, we need to get out of the whirling of your mind and into the present environment around you.

To assist your system in slowing down into the counter-vortex, begin to orient to one sensory channel around you. This either can be something you see, hear, smell, taste, or touch. As you start to notice this sensory input, can you fixate even more on one example? For instance, if you're orienting using your eyes, instead of wandering in the space, can you find one thing to focus on? As you do this, begin to bring your awareness to the intricacies of this visual resource. Can you make out its texture, imperfections, patterns or colors, lines, shadows, or the way the light hits it? Allowing your senses to slow down and sharpen their focus on one thing can support your hyperactive mind.

Anger in the Moment

Anger is a high-energy and mobilizing response that propels us upward and forward—we blow *up*—especially when it shows up out of the blue. It can feel like an out-of-body experience.

To help you ground before gently moving through this anger, start by noticing your feet on the ground. Feel the pressure of your weight in the soles of the feet. Leaning into your vestibular system, shift your weight slowly from right to left, noticing how the large muscles in each leg brace and release as you do so. Start to track what it feels like to be grounded in this moment, to be present. Orient to the space to really deepen this anchor into the counter-vortex.

At Large Gatherings

Large gatherings come with increased stimulation to the body and senses. In a sea of people and commotion, the noise can become quickly overwhelming.

As a resource, try orienting to one particularly pleasant sound. Maybe it's a person whose calming voice you focus on while following the rhythmic variation and inflection of their words. Or perhaps it's the melodic and gentle music playing in the background, which you naturally begin to sway to.

At Work

I encourage you to have a neutral space or a safe haven at your place of work. It should be a place that brings an overall sense of ease, safety, and comfort. This could be your office, a certain room in the building, a bench outside, a particular chair, or even out in your car. When dealing with work stress, can you visit this space to orient for a moment?

Chronic Pain

Pain heightens when we bring more attention to it, and especially when we fear or resist it.

To begin to show your body that it can contain pain, as well as comfort and ease, I invite you to ask the question *Is there a place in my body that feels easier to be with right now?* For many who experience full-body pain, it may start with an area as small as your fingers or toes, or a larger area like your face. Begin to bring awareness to this part of your body, observing through interoception what you might feel in that particular place. It might be easier to use pressure or touch to really feel into this space. As an example, you could tap and press your fingertips together.

Delays

Delays are often unavoidable and out of our control. For this reason, they often can cause our physiology to ramp up as anxiety or frustration takes over.

In these moments, we can help our nervous system slow down and pendulate into the counter-vortex. A supportive resource could be to practice the five-four-three-two-one mindfulness exercise, as you slowly bring awareness to five things you can see, four things you can touch, three things you can hear, two things you can smell, and one thing you can taste.

Digestive Issues

Our nervous system has a bidirectional relationship with our digestive system. When our digestion is off, our nervous system is impacted, and vice versa. For instance, when we're in a sympathetic fight-or-flight response, our digestion is disrupted as blood motility moves away from the gut to flow to the arms and limbs for fighting or fleeing. In essence, when activated, the body conserves energy from other working systems in the body, because it sees survival as priority number one.

Easing tension within the body is one way to support proper digestive function. With this in mind, try tracking an area in your body that feels easiest to focus on. Perhaps it's your feet. As you bring awareness to your feet, try to allow a full stretch from your ankle to your toes—think of the kind of full-bodied stretch we impulsively do when yawning or first waking up. As the stretch releases, bring your attention to the relaxation in your feet and legs. Notice its qualities, and sense into the feeling. This attentional network will show your body and nervous system that they can lean into ease and expansion, rather than tension and contraction.

Feeling Threatened by Strangers

Try imagining that there is a protective force field around you, one that's impenetrable and takes up lots of space. Or imagine that a protective person or figure in your life (or one imagined) is standing between you and this stranger.

Getting Lost

In environments where things feel particularly unfamiliar, you can lean into what is familiar to help yourself resource.

This could include calling a familiar person, looking through the photo album on your phone, listening to a song you've always enjoyed, reflecting on a pleasant memory, orienting to the familiarity of your car that you're currently driving, and more.

In Traffic or on Public Transportation

Kinesthetic orienting is a great way to calm an overwhelmed and overstimulated nervous system. Try orienting to a single object through touch if you feel stressed while commuting or traveling somewhere. Perhaps you can train your attention on the steering wheel, feeling its grooves, texture, temperature, creases, buttons, indents, firmness, or softness. If you're on public transport, perhaps you can feel the texture of your bag, the individual links on your chain necklace, or the softness of your clothes.

Insomnia

When your nervous system is busy running from a tiger, the last thing it wants you to do is rest and digest.

A wonderful resource for insomnia is to slowly tense and relax one body part at a time (known as pandiculation). You can do this while lying flat on your back in your bed. Starting from head to toe, gently begin to stretch and tense your different body parts—neck, shoulders, chest, arms, hands and fingers, stomach, glutes, large leg muscles, calves, feet, and toes. With each stretch, feel into the release and relaxation as you anchor into the counter-vortex. It might help to imagine your body and muscles melting into the bed with each movement.

Medical Anxiety

It's likely that you may have experienced either traumatic illness in the past (being hospitalized, losing a loved one to a sudden medical condition, having a child who became dramatically sick) or some kind of medical trauma. If this is the case, you can use a Somatic Experiencing technique called "T-model" (*T* for *time*) to remind you that there was once safety and wellness to be experienced in the body.

Think of the T-model as a timeline, where T –0 is the traumatic experience, T –10 is the time leading up to the moment, and T +10 is the time following the experience. You can use the T-model as a way to titrate the approach of working directly with a traumatic moment. Rather than diving straight into the traumatic event, by using the T-model, you start by recalling the experience from far in the past, before the trauma occurred, or recalling the experience from in the future, after the trauma occurred, and then move your way inward to T –0, the moment of impact.

With T +10 in mind, can you bring into your mind the season of life after the traumatic illness or medical trauma passed, when you knew everything was going to be okay? Paint a detailed photo in your mind of that time.

If you aren't able to create these images, could you perhaps imagine what life would be like if your health was guaranteed? What does that picture look like? What are you doing, where are you, and who are you with? As always, track through interoception or SIBAM how this feels in the body as you bring this visualization to life.

Obsessive-Compulsive Disorder (OCD)

Keep in mind that OCD often correlates to a chronic flight response. To help address it, you want to intentionally allow the nervous system to slow down so it can gently pendulate and discharge the intense mobilizing hormones of your sympathetic response.

You can do this by grounding your body to the present moment.

Begin to notice the ground below your feet, the chair beneath your sit-bones, or the back of the seat against your back. As you do this, can you welcome in any of these stories: *My body has support, I can rest into this support,* or *My body is grounded and with this support I am sturdy?* As you do this, notice if there is any resting down or easing of the body.

Overwhelm

We are overwhelmed when we're at the tipping point of fight or flight, and about to enter into shutdown, freeze, or dissociation. This is where things often feel like *too much, too fast, too soon.*

Because overwhelm often can be a full-body experience, my suggestion is to look externally for resources that bring you back into your counter-vortex. This could be a moment of co-regulation with a person or pet; it could be noticing the ground or seat below you or allowing your eyes to follow the gentle movement of nature (for example, a bird in the distance, the wind in the trees, a plane flying high overhead, etc.); or it could be the sound of a song playing in the background. Looking outside yourself to concrete evidence that you are grounded and present can be most supportive.

Procrastination

The opposite of procrastination is productivity, performance, and power. Your healthy aggression (from your fight response) and vital life force energy are what propel you to move forward, to go for it, to get stuff done. Yet when you have a nervous system with a limited capacity to be with healthy aggression and power, you instead suppress that life force, placing yourself in procrastination.

Because procrastination occurs in your dorsal shutdown response, you want to first focus on anchoring your body and system into a felt sense of safety and presence, allowing you to "thaw out" so you can then begin to move up the nervous system ladder. Resources that could support you include exposure to temperature (standing in front of an open freezer or cold water on the face or hands), change of environment (sitting outside), co-regulation, supportive self-touch (the Somatic Experiencing self-hug, containment, or muscle massage exercises), or the VOO exercise.

Public Speaking

As a professional speaker of many years who used to struggle with stage fright, here are some of my favorite resources for public speaking. For me, it's the anxiety before the program or presentation that builds up. When this happens, I like to play welcome music in the venue or space. Opt for familiar music that you find comforting or regulating to your system. I have a certain playlist that I've used for more than ten years, for instance. Co-regulating with others directly before an event can be a supportive resource, as it helps your system become familiar with the individuals you'll be talking to. Creating this rapport and social engagement neutralizes the perception that they are strangers or that they're a threat. Can you have a dedicated space before your program to process those anxious nerves? Knowing that you have a space, just for you, can bring ease into your system. Do what you can to ground yourself in your body.

Ruminating Thoughts

You can view ruminating and catastrophic thoughts as not an over-thinking problem, but instead as an underfeeling problem. Because we know that *state creates story*, the goal is not to redirect your thoughts—as you know, that will just add more pressure to the system—but to get out of your head and into your body.

How can you begin to move inward and find resource, relaxation, and refuge? Moving directly into the body may feel foreign and, therefore, overwhelming, so a titrated resource is to practice kinesthetic orienting. Can you hold an object that has sentimental meaning in your hand and begin to examine and observe it? As you do this, what do you notice internally? If going straight to interoception and sensation feels like too much, instead track the layers of SIBAM.

Self-Medicating

People self-medicate as a way to suppress whatever feels like *too much* to be with. You can become numb and dissociated as you enter into states of either shutdown or functional freeze.

From shutdown, you can start by slowly building capacity to be in your body and in the present. Begin to ask yourself *How do I know I'm here in this moment?* The answers could be limitless. Perhaps you feel the seat or ground below you. Perhaps you can lean into the senses of your body as you begin to orient. Perhaps you can conceptualize where you are in space and time.

Unexpected Circumstances or Situations

Sudden change can leave you feeling out of control or fearful of the unknown.

Using visualization, can you begin to imagine the last time you felt in control of a situation, or when something turned out just as you had planned or hoped for? What was that experience like for you? Can you slowly walk yourself through the experience? As you do so, can you notice any easing in your body?

Let the Wild Rumpus Start

I believe not only that trauma is curable, but that the healing process can be a catalyst for profound awakening.
—Peter Levine

My children lie nestled up against me on the bed. My daughter is nine months old now, and my son is nearing four years. I'm reading to them from Maurice Sendak's *Where the Wild Things Are,* a cherished favorite from my own childhood—this inherited copy a link to those bedtime stories my parents once shared with my brothers and me. The book, a simple yet evocative tale, follows Max, a mischievous boy sent to bed without supper. His anger transforms into wild dreams, where he travels across the ocean and becomes king of the Wild Things (symbolizing his untamed emotions) and leads them on a Wild Rumpus of unfiltered expression.

In Sendak's narrative, Max's frustration with his mother is welcomed, magnified, and made flesh in a dreamworld where he can safely explore his emotions, assured of unconditional love upon his return—where supper was waiting for him when he awoke. As I read,

Noah and Shia gleefully reenact the wordless Wild Rumpus, roaring, growling, dancing, and jumping on the bed with unbridled joy.

In this moment, my motherly wish for my children to remain this free and expressive emerges. I take in their faces, and I can't help but wonder what pain they'll endure in their lifetimes. What hard and tormenting lessons life will throw their way. How their hearts will be broken, ripped apart by grief, disappointment, and hurt. It's inevitable in this life. Will they become like the rest of us and tame their wild emotions? Will they mask them behind a thick plate of armor? Or will they know, like Max did, that their uninhibited feelings, no matter how wild, carry with them boundless wisdom and opportunity?

It's ironic, really, how the path to healing unfolds. There is complexity not only to our traumatic experiences but also to the biological structures that house these experiences. And yet, the thing that is the most healing is often the simplest approach. We're realizing now that many healing practices bring us back to a state akin to the original womb-like and childlike seasons of our past—a realm of innocence and exploration, void of self-judgment. Healing often involves reconnecting with our childlike wonder and expression, ultimately returning us to our authentic selves. We do this through embracing silence, play, curiosity, and power, and by immersing ourselves in the natural rhythms of the body and world. It's like *The Curious Case of Benjamin Button*, really—we tumble forward into old age, but at some point, the search for meaning, healing, and self requires that we live backward into infancy. Back into our authentic individuality, rather than our conditioned personality. Back into our nature, rather than our nurture.

I can vividly remember the first time I was able to sit alongside my authentic self. I had just wrapped up a two-month work assignment in India with a grassroots organization fighting to end forced child marriage. I had flown down to the southern state of Kerala, located on the western coast along the Arabian Sea, to decompress and reflect. My grandmother, who had found healing and solace at a local ashram in Kerala following her stroke, was insistent that I visit the ashram and her spiritual teacher before heading home. Of course I agreed. Known for its lush landscapes, wildlife, beautiful beaches, serene backwaters, and world-famous Ayurvedic and yoga centers, it's clear to see why Indians refer to this land as "God's country."

Before heading to the ashram, I spent my first four days in Kerala relaxing in the seaside town of Varkala, where I stayed in an Airbnb owned by a man named Jassar. He had turned his family's beachside coconut farm into a small private resort with three separate villas. It was truly heaven on earth. I spent my days enjoying fresh, delicious, home-cooked food; practicing yoga twice a day next to the ocean; exploring up and down the coast; and slowing down to the rhythm of nature's surroundings.

On the third night, I sat atop the cliff outside my villa overlooking the crashing waves, mesmerized by the setting sun disappearing into the sea. The beauty of the scene laid before me brought on a visceral and emotional reaction that took me by surprise. As if the sun was thawing the frozen residue of my body, my emotions and my sensory channels came back to life. The cyclical sounds of the waves, the vibrant hues that blanketed and reflected upon the water and sand, the smell of salty air, the taste of the fresh coconut I drank out of, the gentle breeze that danced through my hair, the warmth of the sun upon my face—everything became crystal clear.

The deeper I could sense into and through my body, the more intense the emotions became. Gratitude and awe suddenly gave way to suppressed decades-old grief as I became one with the energy and aliveness of the natural world around me. Here I was just like Max, on the other side of the ocean with my very own wild and untamed emotions. It was in this moment that the masks and veils were removed, as reflections of who I was without the titles, the career, the trauma, and the relationships began to form in my mind. I felt bare, exposed, and finally seen and held for the first time. I often reflect on that moment as an awakening, when I realized that the greatest tools to my own healing were already within me, not something I could find outside in a spiritual teacher, a therapist, or a medication. And although those things could be supportive, it turned out that *I was my own best healer.*

Hippocrates said that "Nature itself is the best physician." It's true; nature is the healing balm of this world. Yet modern culture has created a conditioned belief that we are separate from nature, that we should fear it and be ashamed of our *own nature*, including our primal wisdom and expression. What we fail to realize is that *we are nature.* We are the most beautiful and resilient species that nature has created on this planet. The naturalistic approach of Somatic Experiencing, which aims to reconnect us to our innate capacity and instinctual resources for self-healing, provides the evidence of that fact.

From the research of animals in the wild, to the human organism, and even our planet's ecosystems, the lessons we learn from the natural world provide a compass for our own healing and vitality. When we look to world events where nature has been destroyed (like the Chernobyl or the Deepwater Horizon catastrophes, for instance), we can witness that, when left untouched, these ecosystems will always regenerate and come back to life all on their own. It takes time, but they come back, often more adept and resilient than before.

George Carlin once shared, "The planet will be here for a long, long—LONG—time after we're gone, and it will heal itself, it will cleanse itself, because that's what it does. It's a self-correcting system."[1] Our biology, if given proper resources and left undisrupted, is the same. Now this naturalistic approach to healing is not the discovery of new concepts. It's rather translation work, based on ancient wisdom that Earth-honoring and indigenous cultures have known for millennia. Just as we as individuals revert to our formative years to heal, we as a species are being called to follow the same path backward into our history.

I'm jolted to the present as my children playfully pile on top of me, along with the weight of the reality that my babies will inevitability experience pain that only they can heal. I can't save them from their suffering—only they can. Knowing what I know now, both personally and professionally, I believe that my role isn't to shield them from discomfort and adversity, but to stand alongside them and empower them to turn toward it with curiosity, compassion, and courage. My role is to reveal to them that the pain of the past truly never leaves you. But sometimes, the pain can cause you to leave yourself. It can separate you from your body, from your life force, from others, and from the world, both the good in it and the bad.

I'll teach them that avoiding isn't the same thing as processing. And what isn't allowed to be safely felt will only fester within the body and mind. So instead of encouraging my children to suppress their suffering, or to seek external quick fixes, I'll gently lead them back home to themselves. Back to the resilience intricately hardwired into their biology.

I am at the same time comforted in knowing that on the other side of that pain, they will find greater joy and vitality than they've ever experienced. Nature's cycles of expansion and contraction guarantee this simple promise. Darkness follows light. Waves come in and go out. Our breath and our heart pulse. This is what healing requires—space and time to be with both suffering and vitality. With hope in my heart, I'm reminded of the time I spent in South Africa alongside Abina and the contagious joy that exuded from her in the midst of unimaginable adversity. Abina was a living testament of Joseph Campbell's observation that "the joy will burn out the pain."[2]

I see that same limitless joy today from the individuals who venture into this somatic world of healing. The individuals who challenge conventional methods of recovery. The ones who dare to get out of their heads and into their bodies. The ones who recognize that there was never anything wrong with them, that they were never broken and in need of fixing. And that in fact, their body and nervous system knew exactly how to respond to keep them safe in the worst chapters that life has to offer.

Body-First Healing is an encouragement to end the vicious war and resistance we've had against the body's profound wisdom and healing. It's a manual back to ourselves. It's an adopted lifestyle, a way of being and existing and connecting back to our nature—the one we've become so detached from. Nervous system healing is not a quick fix, a last resort, or a hack. The goal is not to make what's hard go away, but to harness greater tools and capacity within your nervous system to withstand the emotional and somatic impacts of your trauma.

As the Wild Rumpus comes to an end, Shia and Noah begin to nuzzle back into me on the bed, energy and emotions expelled. As they settle, I can now feel their soft and calming presence. Rubbing their backs, I catch a glimpse of the small but mighty tattoo on my right wrist: *Infragilis et tenera,* which translates from Latin to "Unbreakable yet tender." I smile and sink my nose into their hair, kissing their foreheads with gratitude. This is the healing and the resilience I get to pass down—both inherited and fought for. My wish for my children, and for this world, is to no longer harden and armor up against life, but to instead soften ourselves to our experiences, allowing our body, our impulses, and our minds to resiliently guide us in the ways they've always known how to do.

My deepest wish is that we all become more like Max. That we learn to face our wild feelings and not tame them. That we "roar our terrible roars," all the while feeling assured that we'll be met with connection, joy, resilience, and vitality.

And with that I'll say, "Let the Wild Rumpus start."

Nervous System Mapping and Tracking

One of the most essential things you can do to make somatic and nervous system healing a regular part of your life is to begin the practice of moving inward, to listen to your body's and physiology's cues. Our body is always speaking to us, whispering through sensations and emotions. Cycles of contraction and expansion present themselves to illustrate where we are within our physiological world. Like learning a new language, it will feel foreign and difficult, and it will take time and repetition to master. At first it will feel forced, but over time it will be fluent. Be sure to utilize the vocabulary of sensation list on page 194 for support.

Here are the steps for daily tracking.

Tracking Your Nervous System

As you become more adept at learning the language of your nervous system, you create more awareness of how your body feels moment to moment.

In the morning:

You will be prioritizing your body, setting one small intention for the day. This is what your *body* wants to accomplish, rather than your brain.

1. Ask yourself this question: *How do I want to* feel *today?*
2. Now identify an emotion. Choose one from the emotional wheel on page 195.
3. Ask yourself how you will accomplish this.

For example, if you want to *feel* playful, you can accomplish this by taking your kids or your dog to a park to run around and be free. Or you could color for a few minutes.

In the evening:

1. Ask yourself this question: *What* felt *pleasant today?*
2. Now identify how your body is showing you (in this moment) that it was pleasant.
3. Reflect on sensations or emotions that come up in the present.

For example, it could be that you got an extra ten minutes to cuddle with your baby and reflecting on how lovely she smells, brings warmness to your chest, and relaxes your shoulders.

These are the kind of questions you can ask:

How am I feeling in my body right now?

What am I noticing about my temperature?

Are my heart and breathing rates elevated?

Do I feel constricted? Do I feel light? Do I feel heavy?

What emotions are present?

Notice and Name

When you notice and name, you will soon become an expert at detecting the state of your nervous system. Practice this once a day for the next week:

- Notice your thoughts, feelings, and the way your body feels.
- Name where you are on the Polyvagal Ladder.
- Get curious. What does your nervous system want you to know in this moment? What's the story it's telling you?

The Polyvagal Triggers and Glimmers Map

Based on the PVT framework, Stephen Porges and Deb Dana developed the Triggers and Glimmers Map (introduced on page 85), which lets you identify what uniquely feels safe (your glimmers) and not safe (your triggers) for your nervous system. Here, for each state, you are going to identify a theme and a specific example of that theme that either triggers you into that response, or regulates you into ventral (your glimmers). For example, if you know that your partner not texting you back triggers a sympathetic fight response, you could ask yourself what the theme is. Perhaps you feel you are being dismissed. You also could start in the reverse order. Maybe you know that feeling out of control triggers you into a sympathetic flight response, and the example you think of is when you're running late somewhere.

Begin the map by first completing your *home-away-from-home* state—that is, your dominant survival state when you're not in ventral. Then, complete your other survival states, ending with the ventral state of safety and connection (your glimmers).

VENTRAL   SAFE AND CONNECTED

Theme:

Example:

Theme:

Example:

Theme:

Example:

SYMPATHETIC   FIGHT OR FLIGHT (3 FOR EACH)

Theme:

Example:

Theme:

Example:

Theme:

Example:

DORSAL   SHUTDOWN

Theme:

Example:

Theme:

Example:

Theme:

Example:

The Polyvagal Personal Profile Map

Based on the PVT framework, Porges and Dana developed the Personal Profile Map (introduced on page 155), which begins the skill of noticing and naming—where you notice a certain emotion, thought, behavior, and somatic cue and can name which state you're in based on that information. This is an important first step in being able to learn the language of your nervous system and to accurately move yourself out of dysregulation. For example, I would never recommend an intense workout to discharge stress hormones if you're in a state of dorsal or shutdown. Therefore, it's important to notice which state you're in before attempting to regulate with a certain tool or practice.

Begin the map by first completing your *home-away-from-home* state—your dominant survival state when you're not in ventral. Then, complete your other survival states, ending with the ventral state of safety and connection (glimmers).

For each of the subsections, aim to identify three to five items. An example is provided below.

VENTRAL	SAFE AND CONNECTED
Somatic:	
Emotions:	
Thoughts:	
Behaviors:	
"I am":	
"The world is":	
Sleep:	
Food:	
Substances:	

Here's an example for ventral:

VENTRAL	SAFE AND CONNECTED
Somatic:	Energized, openness, in the zone, concentrating, present, light, smiling, wanting to move, lifted posture, buzzy
Emotions:	Excited, happy, content, optimistic, positive, playful
Thoughts:	I can do it, too; I'm capable; I'm grateful; I'm lucky
Behaviors:	Expressive, self-care (journaling, meditating, reading), productive, exercising, laughing, social
"I am":	So capable, so successful, happy, living my dream life
"The world is":	A playground full of possibilities
Sleep:	I sleep my average amount
Food:	I eat my average amount
Substances:	Not drawn to any substances (for example, alcohol, drugs, caffeine, or sugar)

SYMPATHETIC	FIGHT OR FLIGHT
Somatic:	
Emotions:	
Thoughts:	
Behaviors:	
"I am":	
"The world is":	
Sleep:	
Food:	
Substances:	

DORSAL	SHUTDOWN
Somatic:	
Emotions:	
Thoughts:	
Behaviors:	
"I am":	
"The world is":	
Sleep:	
Food:	
Substances:	

The Polyvagal Regulating Resources Map

Based on the PVT framework, Porges and Dana developed the Regulating Resources Map (introduced on page 182). As you know, you naturally move up and down the Polyvagal Ladder all day, every day. This map identifies what you need to do to self-regulate or co-regulate. It will help you track your steps.

Begin the map by first completing your *home-away-from-home* state—that is, your dominant survival state when you're not in ventral. Then, complete your other survival state, ending with the ventral state of safety and connection. For each of the three sections, aim to identify five behaviors or practices you'll use to either experience or express from that state to bring you up the ladder. Note that you will be doing two maps total: one for self-regulation, where you identify activities you do alone, and one for co-regulation, where you identify activities you do with another living being. (This can include humans or animals.)

Although you might not start your map in dorsal, let me walk you through the mapping process from bottom to top. At the very bottom of the ladder, when you are in a state of dorsal shutdown, disconnection, rest, and conservation, you'll want to (1) prioritize rest and repair at the very bottom; (2) move up to the middle of dorsal, getting present in your body and in your environment; and (3) at the top of dorsal, bring in light movement to inspire your system to move up into sympathetic fight or flight.

Here are some examples, starting from the very bottom and working your way up:

1. Take a nap.
2. Listen to sad music—honoring where you are.
3. Sit outside, get a breath of fresh air, and connect with nature through the senses.
4. Stretch.
5. Go for a short walk.

Now, you want to gently start to mobilize yourself into a fight-or-flight state. To move from the bottom of a sympathetic state and work your way up, you want to increase the mobilizing energy of the activity so you can begin to express and discharge the adrenaline and cortisol within your body and physiology.

Here are some examples, working from the bottom of sympathetic up to the top of sympathetic on the way to ventral:

1. Do some chores around the house.
2. Go run an errand.
3. Do some light movement like yoga, stretching, or taking a long walk.
4. Allow tears or emotion to flow and be expressed.
5. Go for a workout or a run, or run in place.

Notice any subtle signs of discharge from the body as you express and expel this mobilizing energy (adrenaline and cortisol) through you.

The next stop on the ladder is ventral. When you reach this state, ask yourself, *How can I anchor myself here?* Ventral actually looks very similar to dorsal, because you're anchoring yourself back into a place of parasympathetic rest and digest.

Starting from the bottom of ventral and moving up to the very top of the nervous system ladder, here are some examples:

1. Get out in nature.
2. Listen to your favorite music.
3. Read a book.
4. Do something creative.
5. Lie down for a rest.

You will use the items on your list as substitutions for behaviors you want to change. When you do, instead of maladaptive coping behaviors, you will now have supportive, regulating resources. It will take intention and practice to start to use these resources in the moments of activation.

I suggest practicing these strategies in moments of deactivation, when you feel regulated and neutral. I often recommend setting an alarm morning, midday, and early evening. When that alarm goes off, check in with your body and your nervous system and track where you may be on the ladder in that moment. (This is where your Personal Profile Map can help.) Depending on where you are, take a few intentional minutes to complete the activity.

When you think of your stress physiology like a pressure cooker, in which the pressure builds throughout the day as you experience more stress and activation, how can you proactively lift the lid as a way to avoid exploding or imploding? Using this map is a great way to do that as well as build in new habitual practices that create new neural networks of impulse the next time you're activated. It will look like this: [Alarm goes off.] *Where am I on my ladder right now? Oh, I'm noticing all those characteristics. It looks like I'm actually in a sympathetic state. Well, let me go look at my regulating resources map. What does it say I should do? When I'm here, I'm going to go for a walk. Okay, I'm going on my walk and let's see if I'm still in flight afterward. And if I am, that's okay, because the aim is to gently move up the ladder, not necessarily jump from state to state.*

After you make your map, print it out and keep it on your desk, in your car, at home, or screenshot it to your phone. Some of my clients even make it the background on their phone as a handy reminder that this is their ladder and here are steps they want to be taking. If you're open to sharing it, do so with people who are close to you. David, for instance, knows most of my regulating resources and can share them with me, which can be supportive in moments when I'm activated and not in my rational brain. Like when he lets me know I should get outside in the sun when I'm feeling down (in dorsal), or that I should go for a walk alone when I'm feeling anxious.

Also, you don't need to use every regulating resource. In fact, you might find that you have one or two in each state that become your go-tos, and that's preferable, because it's less remembering and intention for your system. Remember, you're creating new habitual patterns, which takes time and practice.

The Polyvagal Time and Tone Graph

Based on the PVT framework, Porges and Dana developed the Time and Tone Graph. It allows you to see the patterns of how your nervous system operates day to day so you can set your day accordingly.

For example, I wake up very early in the morning ready to go. In this part of the day, I'm toward the top of my nervous system ladder, teetering in a blended state of ventral and sympathetic. I'm productive, creative, and energized—thanks to the extra healthy boost of adrenaline and cortisol. I have moments of solitude that stimulate my creativity. Then, I go for my morning walk for twenty minutes no matter what the weather to get some fresh air. Next up is a bit of at-home exercise, and lastly, I settle into the day with my matcha tea and breakfast. By 5 or 6 p.m., on the other hand, I go down the Polyvagal

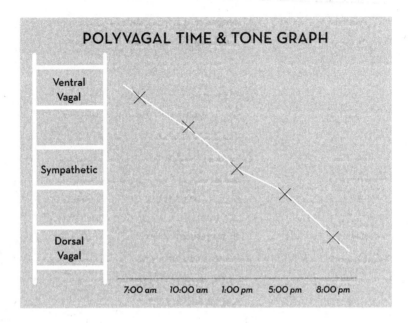

ladder toward dorsal and need rest and solitude. It's safe to say I'm a morning person.

My husband is the complete opposite. He wakes up two hours after I do and it takes him a while to get going. He won't talk in anything more than sighs and nods until he has his coffee. I know not to discuss anything serious with him in the morning. He's most energized when I'm starting to wind down; he's a night owl who prefers afternoon workouts and evening house projects. He's clearly an evening person.

My clients are about half morning and half evening people. Knowing when your system has its peak activation is an important step to cultivating a somatic lifestyle. You always want to work in tandem with your physiology rather than against it.

To begin tracking the daily patterns or "tone" of your nervous system, check in with your nervous system multiple times (three to five) throughout the day and mark on the graph where you're at on the ladder. Make sure to note the time on the X-axis (horizontal) line. Repeat this process for at least two weeks to gauge the overall tone of your nervous system. Use the graph above as a reference to create your own.

How to Find a Somatic Experiencing Practitioner

Those who want to become a Somatic Experiencing Practitioner (SEP™) must complete the three-year professional training program through Somatic Experiencing International that was created by Dr. Peter A. Levine. For more information, go to traumahealing.org. On that site, you can also search for a trained practitioner in your area.

What to Look for in a Somatic Practitioner or Trauma Professional

There are several essential steps you should take before you start your somatic healing journey with a practitioner or therapist:

- You're about to trust someone with some of the most vulnerable aspects of your life—and that's a really big deal. So, I'd recommend against jumping into a therapy chair, or what somatic practitioners call a container, without first completing your research. This includes talking with the practitioner, learning their professional background and experience, and getting a sense for how your system aligns with theirs.

- Because you've already learned about co-regulation in this book, you know that will be an incredibly important part of your therapeutic relationship. If you don't feel safe with your practitioner or your therapist, this will activate your nervous system even more and be counterproductive. SEPs spend quite a bit of time at the beginning of their sessions with new clients building a rapport and ensuring there is a safe and attuned connection to deepen the work. That creates a level of trust and regulation, which is vital for nervous system healing.

- Ask yourself if your practitioner spends time building your capacity, or your ability to be in your body. Or do they keep you strictly in the thought and meaning-making channels of the therapeutic process? Or do they quickly take you out of discomfort anytime it arises? Somatic and nervous system healing require that we move inward on the path to regulation and that we deepen our capacity to be with what feels good and what does not feel good.

- Ask yourself if your practitioner promotes titration. Or do they move in a pace or with content that feels like *too much, too fast, too soon?*

- Does your practitioner give you practices, tools, and exercises for you to work with outside the therapeutic container? It's important that with the aim of self-empowerment and self-healing in mind, you're given encouragement and time to integrate the work into your daily life. This creates a dynamic in which you can begin to trust in your own innate resources, body, and vitality.

APPENDIX C

References

This list references the books, articles, and resources that were cited in *Body-First Healing*. I also included some additional resources for learning more about the topics discussed.

Somatic Experiencing and Trauma

Levine, Peter A. *An Autobiography of Trauma: A Healing Journey*. Rochester, VT: Park Street Press, 2024.

Levine, Peter A. *Healing Trauma: A Pioneering Program for Restoring the Wisdom of Your Body*. Louisville, CO: Sounds True, 2005.

Levine, Peter A. *Trauma and Memory: Brain and Body in a Search for the Living Past; A Practical Guide for Understanding and Working with Traumatic Memory*. Berkeley, CA: North Atlantic Books, 2015.

Levine, Peter A. *Waking the Tiger: Healing Trauma*. Berkeley, CA: North Atlantic Books, 1997.

Levine, Peter A. "Panic, Biology, and Reason: Giving the Body Its Due." *The USA Body Psychotherapy Journal* 2, no. 2 (2003).

Ives, E. "Peter Levine and Somatic Experiencing." *Journal of Psychiatry and Mental Illness* 3, no. 1 (2020): 101.

Campbell, Susan. *From Triggered to Tranquil: How Self-Compassion and Mindful Presence Can Transform Relationship Conflicts and Heal Childhood Wounds*. Novato, CA: New World Library, 2021.

Cook, Alexandra, Joseph Spinazzola, Julian Ford, Cheryl Lanktree, Margaret Blaustein, Marylene Cloitre, Ruth DeRosa, et al. "Complex Trauma in Children and Adolescents." *Psychiatric Annals* 35, no. 5 (2005): 390–398.

Dispenza, Joe, PhD. https://drjoedispenza.com.

Doidge, Norman. *The Brain's Way of Healing: Remarkable Discoveries and Recoveries from the Frontiers of Neuroplasticity.* New York: Penguin Life, 2015.

Epstein, Mark. *The Trauma of Everyday Life.* New York: Penguin Press, 2013.

Fisher, Janina. *Healing the Fragmented Selves of Trauma Survivors: Overcoming Internal Self-Alienation.* Oxfordshire, UK: Routledge, 2017.

Fisher, Janina. *Transforming the Living Legacy of Trauma: A Workbook for Survivors and Therapists.* Eau Claire, WI: PESI Publishing and Media, 2021.

Gordon, Alan, and Ziv Alon. *The Way Out: A Revolutionary, Scientifically Proven Approach to Healing Chronic Pain.* New York: Avery, 2021.

Harris, Nadine Burke. *The Deepest Well: Healing the Long-Term Effects of Childhood Adversity.* Boston: Mariner Books, 2018.

Hawkins, David R. *Healing and Recovery.* London: Hay House, 2015.

Heller, Laurence, and Aline Lapierre. *Healing Developmental Trauma: How Early Trauma Affects Self-Regulation, Self-Image, and the Capacity for Relationship.* Berkeley, CA: North Atlantic Books, 2012.

Hübl, Thomas. *Healing Collective Trauma: A Process for Integrating Our Intergenerational & Cultural Wounds.* Louisville, CO: Sounds True, 2020.

Hyman, Mark, MD. "How Trauma Makes Us Sick And How We Can Heal." Mark Hyman MD. September 14, 2022, https://drhyman.com/blog/2022/09/14/podcast-ep599.

Kardiner, Abram. *The Traumatic Neuroses of War.* Eastford, CT: Martino Fine Books, 2012.

Kennedy, Russell, MD. https://www.theanxietymd.com.

LaPierre, Aline. "A Shaman's Scientific Journey: Conversation with Peter Levine." *International Body Psychotherapy Journal* 19, no. 1 (2020). https://www.ibpj.org/issues/articles/Aline%20LaPierre%20-%20A%20Shamans%20Scientific%20Journey%20Conversation%20with%20Peter%20Levine.pdf.

Lerner, Paul. *Hysterical Men: War, Psychiatry, and the Politics of Trauma in Germany, 1890–1930*. Ithaca, NY: Cornell University Press, 2009.

Maté, Gabor. *The Myth of Normal: Trauma, Illness, and Healing in a Toxic Culture*. New York: Avery, 2022.

Maté, Gabor. *Scattered Minds: A New Look at the Origins and Healing of Attention Deficit Disorder*. Toronto: Knopf Canada, 1999.

Maté, Gabor. *When the Body Says No: Exploring the Stress-Disease Connection*. Wauwatosa, WI: Trade Paper Press, 2011.

Maté, Gabor. *The Wisdom of Trauma*. 2022; Sebastopol, CA: Science & Nonduality. https://thewisdomoftrauma.com.

McConnell, Susan. *Somatic Internal Family Systems Therapy: Awareness, Breath, Resonance, Movement, and Touch in Practice*. Berkeley, CA: North Atlantic Books, 2020.

Menakem, Resmaa. *My Grandmother's Hands: Racialized Trauma and the Pathway to Mending Our Hearts and Bodies*. Las Vegas: Central Recovery Press, 2017.

Moorjani, Anita. *Dying to Be Me: My Journey from Cancer, to near Death, to True Healing*. London: Hay House, 2012.

Neufeld, Gordon, Ph.D. https://neufeldinstitute.org/.

Oldfield, Georgie. *Chronic Pain: Your Key to Recovery*. Huddersfield, UK: Self-published, 2015.

Ozanich, Steven Ray. *The Great Pain Deception: Faulty Medical Advice Is Making Us Worse*. Cardiff by the Sea, CA: Waterside Productions, 2020.

Perry, Bruce D. *Brief: Reflections on Childhood, Trauma and Society*. Houston: The ChildTrauma Academy Press, 2013.

Perry, Bruce D., and Oprah Winfrey. *What Happened to You? Conversations on Trauma, Resilience, and Healing*. New York: Flatiron Books: An Oprah Book, 2021.

Rediger, Jeffrey. *Cured: Strengthen Your Immune System and Heal Your Life*. New York: Flatiron Books, 2020.

Rothschild, Babette, PhD. *The Body Remembers: The Psychophysiology of Trauma and Trauma Treatment*. New York: W. W. Norton, 2000.

Sarno, John E. *The Divided Mind: The Epidemic of Mindbody Disorders.* New York: Harper, 2006.

Sarno, John E. *The Mindbody Prescription: Healing the Body, Healing the Pain.* New York: Grand Central Publishing, 1998.

Schubiner, Howard. *Unlearn Your Anxiety and Depression.* Pleasant Ridge, MI: Mind Body Publishing, 2016.

Schubiner, Howard. *Unlearn Your Pain,* 4th ed. Pleasant Ridge, MI: Mind Body Publishing, 2022.

Schwartz, Richard C., PhD. https://ifs-institute.com/.

Schwartz, Richard, PhD. *No Bad Parts: Healing Trauma and Restoring Wholeness with the Internal Family Systems Model.* Louisville, CO: Sounds True, 2021.

Siegel, Dan, MD. https://drdansiegel.com.

Siegel, Dan, MD. https://heartmindonline.org/resources/daniel-siegel-flipping-your-lid.

Siegel, Daniel J. *The Developing Mind: How Relationships and the Brain Interact to Shape Who We Are,* 3rd ed. New York: Guilford Press, 2020.

Teicher, Martin H., Jacqueline A. Samson, Carl M. Anderson, and Kyoko Ohashi. "The Effects of Childhood Maltreatment on Brain Structure, Function and Connectivity." *Nature Reviews Neuroscience* 17, no. 10 (2016): 652–666.

Tronick, Ed, Isabelle Mueller, Jennifer DiCorcia, Richard Hunter, and Nancy Snidman. "A Caretaker Acute Stress Paradigm: Effects on Behavior and Physiology of Caretaker and Infant." *Developmental Psychobiology* (2020): 1–10.

van der Kolk, Bessel A. *The Body Keeps the Score: Brain, Mind, and Body in the Healing of Trauma.* New York: Viking Press, 2014.

van der Kolk, Bessel A. "The Devastating Effects of Ignoring Child Maltreatment in Psychiatry." *Journal of Child Psychology and Psychiatry* 57, no. 3 (2016): 267–270.

van der Kolk, Bessel A., Julian D. Ford, and Joseph Spinazzola. "Comorbidity of Developmental Trauma Disorder (DTD) and Post-Traumatic Stress Disorder: Findings from the DTD Field Trial." *European Journal of Psychotraumatology* 10, no. 1 (2019): 1562841.

van der Kolk, Bessel A. "Trauma and Memory." *Psychiatry and Clinical Neurosciences* 52, no. S1 (1998): S52–S64. https://doi.org/10.1046/j.1440-1819.1998.0520s5S97.x.

Walker, Pete. *Complex PTSD: From Surviving to Thriving; A Guide and Map for Recovering from Childhood Trauma.* Self-published, 2021.

Wolynn, Mark. *It Didn't Start with You: How Inherited Family Trauma Shapes Who We Are and How to End the Cycle.* New York: Penguin Life, 2016.

Yau, Julie Brown. *The Body Awareness Workbook for Trauma: Release Trauma from Your Body, Find Emotional Balance, and Connect with Your Inner Wisdom.* Oakland, CA: Reveal Press, 2019.

Polyvagal Theory

Dana, Deb. *Polyvagal Exercises for Safety and Connection: 50 Client-Centered Practices.* New York: W. W. Norton, 2020.

Dana, Deb. *The Polyvagal Flip Chart: Understanding the Science of Safety.* New York: W. W. Norton, 2020.

Dana, Deb. *The Polyvagal Theory in Therapy: Engaging the Rhythm of Regulation.* New York: W. W. Norton, 2018.

Porges, Stephen W. *The Polyvagal Theory: Neurophysiological Foundations of Emotions, Attachment, Communication, and Self-regulation.* New York: W. W. Norton, 2011.

Porges, Stephen W., and Senta A. Furman, "The Early Development of the Autonomic Nervous System Provides a Neural Platform for Social Behavior: A Polyvagal Perspective." *Infant and Child Development* 20, no. 1 (2011): 106–118. doi:10.1002/icd.688.

Porges, Stephen W., and Seth Porges. *Our Polyvagal World: How Safety and Trauma Change Us.* New York: W. W. Norton, 2023.

Polyvagal Institute. https://www.polyvagalinstitute.org/.

Attachment

Borg, Lydia K., "Holding, Attaching and Relating: A Theoretical Perspective on Good Enough Therapy Through Analysis of Winnicott's Good Enough Mother, Using Bowlby's Attachment Theory and Relational

Theory." Master's thesis, Smith College, Northampton, MA, 2013. https://scholarworks.smith.edu/theses/588.

Bowlby, John. *Attachment* (2nd ed.). London: Penguin, 1984.

Heller, Diane Poole. *The Power of Attachment: How to Create Deep and Lasting Intimate Relationships.* Louisville, CO: Sounds True, 2019.

Levine, Amir, and Rachel S. F. Heller, *Attached: The New Science of Adult Attachment and How It Can Help You Find—and Keep—Love.* New York: TarcherPerigee, 2010.

Main, Mary, Erik Hesse, and Nancy Kaplan. "Predictability of Attachment Behavior and Representational Processes at 1, 6, and 19 Years of Age: The Berkeley Longitudinal Study." In *Attachment from Infancy to Adulthood: The Major Longitudinal Studies,* edited by Klaus E. Grossman, Karin Grossman, and Everett Waters, 245–304. New York: Guilford Press, 1968.

Main, Mary, Erik Hesse, and Siegfried Hesse. "Attachment Theory and Research: Overview with Suggested Applications to Child Custody." *Family Court Review* 49, no. 3 (2011): 426–463.

Main, Mary, Nancy Kaplan, and Jude Cassidy. "Security in Infancy, Childhood, and Adulthood: A Move to the Level of Representation." *Monographs of the Society for Research in Child Development* 50, no. ½ (1985): 66–104.

Main, Mary, and Judith Solomon. "Discovery of an Insecure-Disorganized/Disoriented Attachment Pattern." In *Affective Development in Infancy,* edited by T. B. Brazelton and M. W. Yogman, 95–124. Norwood, NJ: Ablex, 1986.

Main, Mary, and Judith Solomon. "Procedures for Identifying Infants as Disorganised/Disoriented During the Ainsworth Strange Situation." In *Attachment in the Preschool Years,* edited by M. T. Greenberg, D. Cicchetti, and E. M. Cummings, 121–160. Chicago: University of Chicago Press, 1990.

Main, Mary, and Jackolyn Stadtman. "Infant Response to Rejection of Physical Contact by the Mother: Aggression, Avoidance, and Conflict." *Journal of the American Academy of Child Psychiatry* 20, no. "2 (1981)", 292–307. https://doi.org/10.1016/S0002-7138(09)60990-0.

Maselko, J., L. Kubzansky, L. Lipsitt, et al. "Mother's Affection at 8 Months Predicts Emotional Distress in Adulthood." *Journal of Epidemiology and Community Health* 65, no. 7 (2011): 621–625.

McLeod, Saul. "John Bowlby's Attachment Theory." SimplyPsychology, January 24, 2024, https://www.simplypsychology.org/bowlby.html.

Ogden, Pat, and Janina Fisher. *Sensorimotor Psychotherapy: Interventions for Trauma and Attachment*. New York: W. W. Norton, 2015.

Solomon, Judith, Robbie Duschinsky, Lianne Bakkum, and Carlo Schuengel. "Toward an Architecture of Attachment Disorganization: John Bowlby's Published and Unpublished Reflections." *Clinical Child Psychology and Psychiatry* 22, no. 4 (2017): 539–560. https://doi.org / 10.1177/1359104517721959.

Sroufe, L. Alan. "Attachment and Development: A Prospective, Longitudinal Study from Birth to Adulthood," *Attachment and Human Development* 7, no. 4 (2005): 349–367.

Sroufe, L. Alan, Byron Egeland, Elizabeth A. Carlson, and W. Andrew Collins. *The Development of the Person: The Minnesota Study of Risk and Adaptation from Birth to Adulthood*. New York: Guilford Press, 2009.

Sroufe, L. Alan. "The Place of Development in Developmental Psychopathology." In *Multilevel Dynamics in Developmental Psychopathology: Pathways to the Future*, edited by Ann S. Masten, 285–299. Mahwah, NJ: Lawrence Erlbaum Associates, 2007. edited by Ann S. Masten, 285–299. Mahwah, NJ: Lawrence Erlbaum Associates, 2007.

van Rosmalen, Lenny, René van der Veer, and Frank van der Horst. "Ainsworth's Strange Situation Procedure: The Origin of an Instrument." *Journal of the History of the Behavioral Sciences* 51, no. 3 (2015): 261–284.

Wallin, David J., *Attachment in Psychotherapy*. New York: Guilford Press, 2007.

ACKNOWLEDGMENTS

This book journey predates the creation of these chapters. It was a collective effort, contributed to by many, over countless years. From emotional support, to mentorship, to expert guidance, and encouragement—I would like to express my deepest gratitude to everyone who supported me throughout this process.

Thank you to my family; your unwavering support and belief in me made this book possible. To my mentors and colleagues, your wisdom, guidance, and nurturing have been instrumental in shaping this book. To my book team, whose dedication and inspiration helped bring this project to life—thank you for making this dream a reality.

In recognizing that I stand on the shoulders of giants, my heartfelt appreciation and awe go out to Dr. Peter A. Levine (the developer of Somatic Experiencing) and Dr. Stephen W. Porges (the developer of the Polyvagal Theory) for their lifelong dedication to body-based approaches to healing. For without your pioneering knowledge, these words and chapters wouldn't exist. To the Somatic Experiencing community at large, including Somatic Experiencing International and the mentors who guided me along the way, in particular Dr. Glyndie Nickerson, Dr. Abi Blakeslee, and Dr. Raja Salvem, thank you for your passion to nurture and lead the next generation of practitioners, and spread the impact of SE worldwide.

Thank you, Karen Murgolo, for being the first to believe in my mission and my message, for being the compass I needed as I navigated becoming a debut author, and for answering my many phone calls, of course. Karen Moline, for shaping and sharpening my words, for bringing joy to this process, and for being the loudest cheerleader in the room. To Lucia Watson, whose careful editing and support made *Body-First Healing* better than I could have ever imagined, and whose direction empowered each page all while letting me be free in my vision. For each individual at Avery Publishing and Penguin Publishing Group who fiercely dedicated themselves to this book's creation, delivery, and impact: Lindsay Gordon, Farin Schlussel, Casey Maloney, Carla Iannone, Jamie Lescht, Isabel Mccarty, Maya Ono, Zehra Kayi, Stephanie Bowen, and Rachael Perriello Henry. And to Caroline Sutton, for so passionately believing in this book from the beginning, for bringing humanness to this project, and for advocating and championing it across the finish line—I am deeply indebted.

To the Healing Hub team, the smallest but mightiest group of inspiring women, thank you for your encouragement, your friendship, and your profound commitment to this work, to our mission, and to our community. Special thank you to Julia Thompson; without your uplifting and loving support, your creative guidance, and your steadfast dedication to our members and our impact, this book wouldn't exist. I'm beyond grateful for you, and everything you do.

To my parents, Stephanie and Alan, it's not lost on me the sacrifices you made to give us the best possible life; thank you. Thank you for modeling what perseverance in the face of immeasurable suffering looks like. Thank you for loving me and empowering me through the hardest seasons of life, for reminding me I am more than what I've been through, and for laying a path of determination and resilience at my feet. I love you. To my brothers, Dominic and Ryan, I love and cherish you both. Thank you for making me the proudest sister.

To my aunt, Nini, thank you for your nurturing spirit, for your kind heart and friendship over all these years. To the rest of my family, thank you for always being present, uplifting, and loving. I'm so proud of where I come from.

To my children, Noah and Shia, for the infinite love we share, for your wild and free spirits, for the opportunity to experience child-hood again alongside you. I hope these stories and chapters bring clarity and comfort. Thank you for gifting me the greatest role in life. I love you my babies.

To my husband, David, for whom I owe the most gratitude. Over fourteen years, your compassionate and loving support, your spiritual stewardship, and your persistent encouragement and guidance have helped shape me into the person I am today. Thank you for loving me, even when I found it hard to love myself. Thank you for believing in me, despite my self-doubts. Thank you for making this life possible for all of us. I love you.

NOTES

Chapter 1: Healing with a Body-First Approach

1. Aline LaPierre, "A Shaman's Scientific Journey: Conversation with Peter Levine," *International Body Psychotherapy Journal* 19, no. 1 (2020): 15–22, https://www.ibpj.org/issues/articles/Aline%20LaPierre%20-%20A%20Shamans%20Scientific%20Journey%20Conversation%20with%20Peter%20Levine.pdf.

2. "New CDC Data Illuminate Youth Mental Health Threats During the COVID-19 Pandemic," CDC Newsroom, March 31, 2022, https://www.cdc.gov/media/releases/2022/p0331-youth-mental-health-covid-19.html.

3. Cynthia L. Lancaster, Daniel F. Gros, Michael C. Mullarkey, Christal L. Badour, Therese K. Killeen, Kathleen T. Brady, and Sudie E. Back, "Does Trauma-Focused Exposure Therapy Exacerbate Symptoms among Patients with Comorbid PTSD and Substance Use Disorders?" *Behavioural and Cognitive Psychotherapy* 48, no. 1 (2020): 38–53.

Chapter 2: The Top-Down and Bottom-Up Approaches for Trauma

1. Gardiner Morse, "Hidden Minds: 95 Percent of Our Brain's Activity Is Subconscious," *Harvard Business Review*, June 2022, https://hbr.org/2002/06/hidden-minds.

2. Emma Wager, Matthew McGough, Shameek Rakshit, Krutika Amin, and Cynthia Cox, "How Does Health Spending in the U.S. Compare to Other Countries?" Health System Tracker, January 23, 2024, https://

www.healthsystemtracker.org/chart-collection/health-spending-u-s
-compare-countries.

Chapter 3: Defining Trauma

1. "Man Faces Rape, Robbery Charges | Wthr.Com," 13WTHR, April 6, 2009, https://www.wthr.com/article/news/local/man-faces-rape-robbery -charges/531-ed61ed1f-12dd-4807-8f0c-33708842a4e0.

2. "Mice Can Inherit Learned Sensitivity to Smell," Emory News Center, January 16, 2014, https://news.emory.edu/stories/2014/01/video_mice _inheriting_sensitivity_to_smell/index.html.

3. Rachel Yehuda, Nikolaos P. Daskalakis, Linda M. Bierer, Heather N. Bader, Torsten Klengel, Florian Holsboer, et. al., "Holocaust Exposure Induced Intergenerational Effects on *FKBP5* Methylation," *Biological Psychiatry* 80, no. 5 (2016), https://doi.org/10.1016/j.biopsych.2015.08.005.

4. "About Adverse Childhood Experiences," CDC, May 16, 2024, https:// www.cdc.gov/aces/about/index.html.

5. Sarah N. Back, Aleya Flechsenhar, Katja Bertsch, and Max Zettl, "Childhood Traumatic Experiences and Dimensional Models of Personality Disorder in DSM-5 and ICD-11: Opportunities and Challenges," *Current Psychiatry Reports* 23, no. 9 (2021): 60.

Chapter 4: Traumatic Memory

1. Pierre Janet, "Essay of Experimental Psychology on the Lower Forms of Human Activity," in *Psychological Automatism*, edited by Félix Alcan, 4th ed., Paris: Ancienne librairie Germer Baillière et Cie, 1903.

2. Mariana Moscovich, Danny Estupinan, Muhammad Qureshi, and Michael S. Okun, "Shell Shock: Psychogenic Gait and Other Movement Disorders—A Film Review," *Tremor and Other Hyperkinetic Movements* 3 (2013).

Chapter 6: How Your Childhood Attachment Informs Your Relationships

1. Gordon Neufeld, "The Keys to Well-Being in Children and Youth," Address, November 13, 2012, https://neufeldinstitute.org/wp-content/uploads/2017/12/Neufeld_Brussels_address.pdf.

2. "Everything You Need to Know About Secure Attachment," *Raised Good*, n.d., https://raisedgood.com/everything-you-need-to-know-about-secure-attachment.

Chapter 7: The Armor of Trauma and the Five Stuck Personalities

1. "Gabor Mate: Attachment and Authenticity Are Basic Needs," INTP Forum, July 24, 2022, https://www.intpforum.com/threads/gabor-mate-attachment-and-authenticity-are-basic-needs.29091/.

2. "Shonda Rhimes '91 Delivers a Lesson-Packed Commencement Address," Dartmouth, June 9, 2014, https://home.dartmouth.edu/news/2014/06/shonda-rhimes-91-delivers-lesson-packed-commencement-address.

Chapter 8: Healthy Aggression and Life Force: Raising Your Power

1. Laurie Udesky, "The Wisdom of Trauma: Gabor Maté, Peter Levine in Conversation about How the Body Heals from Trauma," California PACEs Action (CA), June 23, 2021, https://www.pacesconnection.com/g/california-aces-action/blog/the-wisdom-of-trauma-gabor-mate-peter-levine-in-conversation-about-how-the-body-heals-from-trauma.

Chapter 9: Somatic Experiencing Basics

1. Brené Brown, *The Gift of Imperfection*, 10th anniversary ed. (New York: Random House, 2020).

Conclusion: Let the Wild Rumpus Start

1. "George Carlin: Saving the Planet – Full Transcript." Scraps from the Loft, August 22, 2019. https://scrapsfromtheloft.com/comedy/george-carlin-saving-planet-transcript/.

2. "17 Inspirational Joseph Campbell Quotes on Success and Following Your Bliss," Inc., October 15, 2018, https://www.inc.com/peter-economy/17-inspirational-joseph-campbell-quotes-on-success-following-your-bliss.html.

INDEX